natural
health
for women

Beth MacEoin

natural
health
for women

Self-help and complementary treatments for more than 100 ailments

hamlyn

First published in Great Britain in 2005
by Hamlyn, a division of Octopus
Publishing Group Ltd
2–4 Heron Quays, London E14 4JP

Distributed in the United States and Canada by
Sterling Publishing Co., Inc.
387 Park Avenue South, New York, NY 10016–8810

ISBN 0 600 61094 2
EAN 9780600610946

A CIP catalogue record for this book
is available from the British Library

Printed and bound in China

10 9 8 7 6 5 4 3 2 1

This book is not intended as an alternative to personal medical advice.
The reader should consult a physician in all matters relating to health and
particularly in respect of any symptoms which may require diagnosis or
medical attention. While the advice and information are believed to be
accurate and true at the time of going to press, neither the author nor the
publisher can accept any legal responsibility or liability for any errors or
omissions that may have been made.

contents

the holistic approach to health

As their lives become increasingly busy and demanding, women find themselves regularly juggling roles of professional worker, mother, partner and carer. Such a challenging lifestyle can place a great strain on the body, leaving it vulnerable to a variety of disorders, so it is not surprising that women are eager for information on how best to maintain their health. Interestingly, much of the information to which they turn relates to complementary therapies.

This interest in complementary and alternative therapies becomes apparent when you flick through the pages of any women's glossy magazine. Almost without exception, any article about a health problem and its treatment by conventional medicine also features a discussion of the complementary approach.

Definitions

• **Holistic** is a term derived from the Greek word *holos*, meaning 'whole', so holistic therapies treat the whole person, rather than just the illness.

• **Alternative medicine** is the practice of medicine without the use of drugs.

• **Complementary medicine** is the practice of medicine that combines traditional and alternative medicine.

the conventional approach

The sophisticated diagnostic techniques now available mean that conventional medicine is very successful at identifying health problems. It also has an impressive repertoire of drugs, painkillers, anesthetics and surgical procedures to call upon.

However, there are downsides. There is a tendency in conventional medicine to compartmentalize health problems into various specialities, such as endocrinology, neurology or gynecology. As a result, although individual practitioners are experts in their own field, they tend to focus on the specific problem rather than seeing it in the context of the whole patient. Conventional medicine is therefore not so successful at dealing with health problems that do not fit into a convenient category, such as auto-immune problems or chronic health conditions. For example, the best that can be done for eczema is to keep the symptoms at bay by using long-term medication.

In addition, any treatment, whether it involves drugs or surgery, has side-effects as well as benefits, and these side-effects can be far-reaching. Antibiotics are a prime example of this. Although their use is sometimes unavoidable, their over-use has led to the emergence of resistant infections such as the MRSA 'superbug' (methicillin-resistant *Staphyloccus aureus*).

the complementary approach

Complementary treatments work from a broader, more ambitious basis, with the aim of gently but effectively supporting or restoring the self-regulating, self-balancing capacity of the body. Any treatment begins with the therapist establishing an overall picture of the patient by asking about the background and lifestyle, eating and drinking habits, exercise, general health and so on.

Most treatments are designed to strengthen the body's immune system so that it is better able to fight illness and infection. Once there is evidence of this happening, no further treatment is necessary. This is because, rather than temporarily suppressing the symptoms of a condition, the treatment addresses the cause of the problem – the imbalance – at source.

Once a condition improves, a patient should feel not only better but also more energized and fitter. This feeling of being truly well is a positive rather than a neutral state. It is not merely being symptom-free but a new state of well-being.

why the natural approach appeals to women

Many women have become disillusioned with conventional medicine because of its compartmental nature. For example, you may be sent to an endocrinologist for hormonal problems, a gynecologist for period problems, a neurologist for tension headaches and migraines, and a gastric specialist for stubborn symptoms of irritable bowel syndrome. The spin-off is that no one takes an overall view of the patient and so the common factor in the conditions, in this case stress, is overlooked. This is where a consultation with a complementary therapist can seem like a breath of fresh air: for many women this is the first time anyone presents them with the whole picture.

Other women are understandably reluctant to take drugs in any form, especially in the long term, because of the potential side-effects and because drugs often address the symptoms rather than the root cause of a problem. They also recognize that there is more to health than an absence of illness, which is exactly what holistic approaches try to achieve.

Before embarking on any form of complementary treatment, it makes sense to give yourself a head start on the road to positive health by making some positive lifestyle changes. Two of the best ways of doing this are to follow a healthier diet, take more exercise and to learn how to rest and relax.

a healthy diet

There a lot of truth in the phrase 'we are what we eat'. A diet of junk foods washed down with sugary or caffeinated drinks or excessive amounts of alcohol is almost certain to cause health problems. It's also likely to cause a lack of energy and vitality as well as making you more prone to recurrent minor infections. Eating regular portions of foods from the groups listed below will ensure you get enough vitamins and minerals.

Wholegrains Eat as many wholegrain foods as possible in the form of brown rice and wholegrain cereals. These have not been stripped of their fibre and nutrients and therefore have more nutritional benefit than the refined varieties.

Fruit and vegetables Include a minimum of five portions of fresh fruit and vegetables each day. These provide antioxidant nutrients which boost the immune system, fight infection and discourage degenerative heart and circulatory disease.

Dairy foods Eat dairy foods in moderation and opt for organic produce whenever you have the opportunity in order to reduce the risk of ingesting synthetic hormones and growth enhancers found in factory-farmed produce.

Fish Include portions of fish regularly, especially oily fish such as mackerel and sardines. These are an excellent source of essential fatty acids that benefit the heart and circulatory system.

Meat Eat red meat only occasionally, as it is high in saturated fat. If you have a craving for red meat, opt for poultry instead.

Once you establish these boundaries, you can enjoy the benefits of a naturally high-fibre, medium-fat, low-sugar and low-salt diet. These rules may sound obvious but, if you stick to them, you will find that your energy levels become more stable, your mood, will be less likely to fluctuate, and your weight should begin to stabilize at a healthy level. Above all, avoid any crash or extreme diets since they do not appear to solve weight problems in the long run and can often leave you nutritionally compromised.

water

Drinking plenty of water is one of the most basic things you can do to keep healthy as it maintains the skin quality and guards against headaches and constipation. Ideally you should drink five large glasses of water each day. Don t rely on feeling thirsty as a guide: by this time you are probably already mildly dehydrated.

Approach with caution!

Convenience foods Avoid take-away meals and unhealthy snacks as these are often high in fat, salt and sugar.

Sugar Avoid foods that contain large amounts of refined white sugar, which can lead to obesity and diabetes. Watch out for hidden sugars in pre-prepared foods.

Salt Too much salt can lead to high blood pressure and heart disease, so use it in moderation.

Fats Saturated fats can raise your cholesterol levels and lead to heart disease. Use unsaturated fats, such as olive, sunflower or safflower oils, wherever possible.

Caffeine Limit your intake of caffeinated drinks, such as tea, coffee and some carbonated drinks, to two cups a day.

Alcohol Limit your weekly intake of alcohol to 14 units (1 unit is equivalent to a glass of wine, a measure of spirits or half a pint of beer). Too much alcohol puts a strain on the liver and increases the risk of addiction and liver disease.

exercise

Before embarking on any exercise plan, it is important to decide what you are trying to achieve: weight loss, greater strength or stamina, more flexibility or general all-round fitness? Also, if you are unused to regular exercise or have some underlying health problem, it may be wise to consult your doctor first. Remember that even walking is of tremendous benefit – the important thing is to keep moving.

types of exercise

Any form of exercise has positive health benefits but some exercises may be better than others if you have a particular goal in mind. If you like the motivation of going to a class, choose systems of exercise such as Pilates, yoga or a class that provides a good cross-section of aerobic work as well as a combination of Pilates and yoga. Don't be misled into thinking that getting fit means investing in the latest stretchy outfit and heading for the gym. Walking has been shown to be one of the most beneficial of exercises for the heart and lungs, as well as working the large muscles of the legs. All you need to do is invest in a good pair of shoes that support the foot and get moving.

Walking, running, swimming and dancing are good all-round activities requiring no special equipment and they all improve stamina and strength to some degree.

Sports and aerobics improve stamina but improvements in strength may be limited to particular muscles. Racquet sports in particular improve balance and coordination.

Weight training can be targeted at particular muscles and can be helpful in improving any weakness, for example after injury.

Yoga, Pilates and tai chi will improve flexibility as well as teaching relaxation and breathing techniques (see pages 56–60).

planning your exercise

There are some simple rules to follow if you want draw up an exercise plan that will really work for you.

• Choose a form of exercise that you will enjoy. Do not necessarily opt for the obvious. With a little thought and imagination, you are more likely to find something that suits you.

• Be realistic about your level of fitness and resist the temptation to take on more than your body can handle.

• Set aside regular times each week for your chosen exercise. To start with this may be three periods of fifteen minutes a week. The best time to exercise is always on an empty stomach in order to avoid cramps and digestive discomfort, ideally avoiding the late evening when it's time to wind down in preparation for a night's rest. As your level of fitness improves, you can either spend longer on the same exercises or you can set yourself more strenuous targets. Whatever you decide, be sure that you can keep to your schedule.

Be patient. In time, if you exercise regularly, you will develop greater strength, stamina and flexibility – and any weight loss will be a bonus!

rest and relaxation

Many problems are directly or indirectly caused by stress, so sleep and relaxation are a priority. Any relaxation technique needs to be a positive, pro-active choice, rather than simply collapsing in front of the television in the hope that will do the trick. The irony is that watching television is more likely to make us stressed, especially if we're watching a really suspenseful programme that's got us on the edge of our seats!

the importance of sleep

A regular, refreshing sleep pattern brings an impressive number of health benefits. These include greater mental clarity and focus, steady levels of energy and vitality, more balanced emotions and an improved ability to fight off minor infections. Ironically, the need for sound sleep increases if you are under severe or extended negative stress, so make a point of getting some early nights rather than burning the candle at both ends. Your body will thank you for it!

relaxation techniques

These are vital tools in helping us deal with the negative stresses that hit us every day. There is a wide choice of techniques.

Meditation Enjoyed every day this has been shown to improve concentration and mental focus, while also lowering blood pressure and reducing stress-related symptoms.

Autogenic training A system of deep relaxation which can relax body and mind.

Progressive muscular relaxation A systematic way of learning how to focus on specific muscle groups by tightening them and letting them go and relax. As a result, this can be used to relax areas of the body that are especially subject to tension.

Yoga A very effective way of combining a relaxing or energizing physical work-out with controlled breathing techniques.

breathing techniques

Controlled breathing aids relaxation. Breathe in slowly, filling your lungs to their full capacity. Then breathe out equally slowly, trying to make the in-breaths equal the out-breaths. To check that you are doing this correctly, place one hand lightly at the base of your chest, just above the navel. Your hand should lift slightly upwards and outwards as you breathe in and return to position when you breathe out. Learning how to breathe in a full, rhythmical relaxed way is an essential part of yoga practice in order to get the maximum benefit from the postures. Mastering controlled breathing techniques is also an integral part of learning tai chi.

health checks

You can take positive steps to look after your health by making sure you have regular health checks and screenings. The following checklist should be helpful. This is not intended to be an exhaustive list, but should give a general idea of some of the routine tests that can be helpful in picking up any potential health problems at an early stage. In many ways, this can be regarded as the best preventative medicine of all, since the sooner a problem can be picked up, the more positive the outcome is likely to be.

Breasts By examining your breasts you should notice any significant changes. Seek medical advice if you notice:

• Puckering of the skin

• Any sign of a lump in the breast or armpit

• Changes in appearance of the nipple or any discharge.

In the UK, women between the ages of 50 and 53, are invited for a mammogram, followed by an annual mammogram for more than 10 years. In other countries, such as the US and Australia, it is recommended that women over the age of 50 should be screened every one to two years.

Cervical smears If you are between 21 and 64 years old, it is advisable to have a smear at least every 3 years.

Blood pressure If you are taking hormone replacement therapy, you should have your blood pressure checked every 3 months or every 6 months if you are taking the contraceptive pill.

Blood Samples can be tested to check blood sugar levels (especially important if you are sedentary, overweight and are worried about heart disease or strokes), cholesterol levels or thyroid function. A blood count can also reveal problems with iron deficiency anaemia. This can be important for women who experience heavy, flooding periods.

Weight It is often better to rely on your own judgement rather than slavishly following height and weight tables. However, if you answer 'yes' to most of the questions in the box, it is time to embark on a sensible weight loss plan.

Skin The texture, tone and quality of your skin can reveal a great deal about your overall health and vitality. Changes in texture or appearance (such as the emergence of moles or any other raised, discoloured patches of skin) should be checked by a doctor. Avoid unprotected exposure to the sun when its effect is at its strongest and use protective creams on exposed areas. Wearing a hat will protect the scalp and the back of the neck.

Smoking Apart from cancer, smoking causes heart disease, hardening of the arteries, the build-up of fatty deposits in the arteries, making us more prone to high blood pressure, and increases the risk of bronchitis, smoker's cough and emphysema.

Are you overweight?

• Do you get breathless when climbing a moderate flight or stairs or walking briskly?

• Do you find it difficult to maintain a conversation when walking with a partner?

• Have you noticed any areas of excess weight on your upper arms, hips, thighs or belly?

• Does your clothing feel uncomfortably tight shortly after you have put it on?

• Do you have trouble regaining your breath after a short spurt of running?

Warning: 'Yes' answers to the first two questions may suggest a heart problem.

seeking professional advice

There are some situations that need the attention of a trained complementary therapist and others that need conventional medical advice or treatment – here are some basic guidelines. Usually, the severity of a condition, the length of its duration and the existence or not of a conventional regime of treatment offers a guide to whether it's suitable for self-help or whether professional complementary treatment is required.

situations for a complementary therapist

Chronic conditions The word chronic does not refer to the severity of the symptoms, but to the established nature of the problem. Chronic conditions, such as arthritis, eczema, premenstrual syndrome and migraine, tend to be well-established and subject to periodic flare-ups. Because the management of these conditions can be difficult, it is best to consult an experienced practitioner.

Acute conditions These problems, such as hangovers, minor injuries and colds, tend to be short-lived. However, if they show signs of getting significantly worse, rather than responding to self-help measures, consult a trained practitioner.

Mixing medicines Most complementary medicines can be used alongside existing conventional drugs but in some cases (such as herbal remedies) they may interact unfavourably. These are discussed in the text.

situations for a doctor

Unusual or serious symptoms These should always be reported to your doctor. If symptoms become serious or life-threatening, this is often a matter of urgency.

Uncertainty If in doubt, always seek medical advice, especially if you fall into an extra-vulnerable category, for example if you are pregnant or elderly.

Mixing medicines If you intend to take complementary medicines as well as conventional drugs, you should discuss this with your doctor beforehand.
Warning On no account stop taking prescribed medicines without consulting your doctor as this can be dangerous.

how to use this book

This book covers the range of complementary therapies available and how to use them. As well as hints and tips about how to select and use complementary medicines, there is also advice on lifestyle changes to improve your health and vitality. It aims to provide some basic tools you can use to stimulate a sense of positive health which will ultimately be more rewarding than being content with symptom suppression.

The complementary therapies featured in this book have been chosen with a view to covering the most comprehensive systems of healing that are suitable for treating a range of acute and/or chronic health problems.

Eastern therapies These can be used to treat a broad range of chronic problems, including skin conditions such as eczema and psoriasis, as well as stress-related conditions, digestive problems and hormonal and reproductive disorders.

Manipulative therapies These are used to treat tension, or back or joint problems.

Natural therapies (See Eastern therapies, above.)

Active and creative therapies (for those wishing to play a more active role, or with an interest in exercise and relaxation).

This information should help you to decide what therapy is best for you. In addition, there is a comprehensive section devoted to ailments, their symptoms and their conventional and complementary treatments. Some require treatment from a skilled practitioner of a complementary therapy, but others may benefit from the simple self-help measures suggested.

Finally there is a first-aid section, which outlines some simple complementary treatments for minor ailments and injuries. A list of warning symptoms indicates whether the problem is serious, or even life-threatening, and therefore requires medical advice.

guidelines for self-treatment

• Always use a reputable supplier when buying over-the-counter complementary medicines and do not be afraid to ask for advice.

• Read the instructions carefully and always follow the recommended dose.

• If in doubt, check that they belong to a recognized register, that they are covered by professional indemnity insurance and are required to abide by a code of ethics and practice.

A home medicine chest of natural remedies

Topical preparations

Aloe vera gel (herbal)

Arnica cream (herbal)

Calendula cream and calendula tincture (herbal)

Lavender essential oil (aromatherapy)

Tea tree essential oil (aromatherapy)

Remedies to be taken internally, with recommended dosage

Aconite (6c) (homoeopathy)

Arnica (6c) (homoeopathy)

Gelsemium (6c) (homoeopathy)

Echinacea tincture (herabal)

Ignatia (6c) (homoeopathy)

Nux vomica (6c) (homoeopathy)

Slippery elm powder or tablets (herbal)

Rescue remedy tincture or spray (flower essence)

complementary therapies

introduction

The common feature of natural therapies is the 'whole body' approach, which regards illness as a sign of imbalance in the systems of the body. Therefore, rather than treating symptoms in isolation, they aim to stimulate the body's natural healing properties by restoring harmony to these systems. They can also be used in the absence of illness to promote extremely positive feelings of good health.

The basis of Eastern therapies is the concept of energy flowing around the body through channels. These channels sometimes become blocked and the aim is to unblock them. This approach is found in acupuncture, acupressure, ayurveda and shiatsu, in exercise systems such as yoga and tai chi, and in reflexology.

Chiropractic and osteopathy aim to restore the physical balance of the body by manipulation of the spine and this, in turn, enables the body's systems to work efficiently. The Alexander technique has much in common with this approach.

The body may need more specific support to cope with a particular ailment, which is where aromatherapy, homeopathy, Bach flower remedies and Chinese and Western herbalism come into their own. Naturopathy and nutritional therapy also have much sensible advice to offer, especially about positive lifestyle changes.

For the more practically inclined, there are the relaxation and exercise techniques described under Creative therapies. These are best learned from a qualified teacher, after which they can be practised alone. Others may benefit from crystal and colour therapies, spiritual healing or arts therapies.

contents

eastern therapies

acupuncture

This well-known complementary therapy has a particularly good track record in providing pain relief for a range of chronic problems, such as lower back pain and chronic headache. Although earlier controlled trials of acupuncture met with some criticism, a sufficient number of double-blind trials have since shown significant positive benefits. This suggests that acupuncture can indeed help reduce the need for pain-killers, especially if the treatment is tailored to the individual patient, rather than a routine treatment that uses the same acupuncture points irrespective of symptoms.

the first treatment

Your acupuncturist will devote a great deal of time to observing you, as well as taking a detailed medical history. Much of the observation revolves around examining your tongue and feeling your pulse, since both are thought to reveal a great deal about the overall health of a patient. Once he or she has made a diagnosis, your acupuncturist can begin treatment. This involves the insertion of extremely fine needles into specific points on your body with the aim of restoring the balance of the chi (vital energy) that is believed to be responsible for good health.

Because the needles are so fine, you should experience no pain or distress on insertion, just a mild tingling; nor is there any bleeding when the acupuncturist removes them. Although patients differ in the sensations they experience and their response to treatment, they all describe a tingling, a slight ache and a sensation of warmth flowing along the part of the body being treated.

Once the needles are in place (usually 15–30 minutes, depending on the acupuncturist's assessment), any initial sensations should subside. If extra stimulation is necessary, the acupuncturist may rotate the needles, apply a tiny current of electricity, or place a smouldering herbal cone of moxa (*Artemesia vulgaris*) at the tip of the needle which will provide a warming sensation.

At the end of the treatment, your acupuncturist may give you some basic advice about activities that you should avoid immediately afterwards. These include strenuous activity, love-making, or eating a heavy meal, all of which place an extra strain on the body.

how does acupuncture work?

There is no definitive explanation of how acupuncture works although there are some tentative theories. One of the main advances was the observation that acupuncture points are areas where there is a perceptible increase in electrical activity and a lowered resistance of the skin. More significantly, the insertion of acupuncture needles at specific points on the body stimulates the production of endorphins. These chemicals, naturally produced by the body, have significant pain-relieving and antidepressant effects.

An acupuncturist works from the basic premise that ill health emerges when there is an imbalance of vital energy, or chi. Conversely, if this vital energy can be stimulated to flow in a balanced way again, good health will emerge once again.

From an acupuncturist's point of view, the internal and external parts of the body are connected by invisible tracks, called meridians, which are located beneath the surface of the skin. These meridians are believed to be the pathways along which the chi travels as it helps maintain optimum levels of mental, emotional and physical health and energy.

Uses of acupuncture

When considering acupuncture as a treatment option, bear in mind that the World Health Organization has identified more than 40 conditions which appear to respond favourably to acupuncture. These include asthma, high blood pressure, insomnia, anxiety, pre-menstrual syndrome, irregular and painful periods. Therefore, this therapy offers much more than just pain relief.

acupressure

Acupressure is an extremely 'hands-on' therapy that utilizes acupuncture points in order to balance and/or stimulate the flow of vital energy, or chi, throughout the body. To do this, the practitioner applies pressure, with hands or feet, to specific points of the body.

Regarded as part of traditional Chinese medicine, acupressure is used in combination with dietary advice, breathing techniques and Chinese herbs in an attempt to give the body the support it needs to get into optimum balance. It can be especially useful in reducing muscle tension and stress-related symptoms.

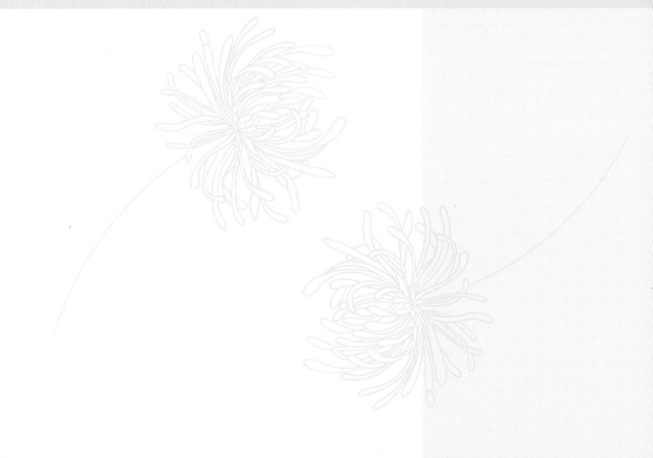

the first treatment

The practitioner will begin by taking a case history and questioning you about general aspects of your lifestyle and diet, the amount of exercise you take and how much stress you have to deal with regularly. They may want to take your pulse, because this is thought to reveal a great deal about your overall state of health.

During the treatment you either lie fully dressed on a firm, comfortable surface (such as a futon), or remain seated. When attending a session, it is a good idea to wear loose-fitting clothes, so that you feel as comfortable as possible throughout the treatment.

Do not be surprised if your practitioner uses a variety of different pressures during a treatment, because the pressure they apply will depend on your individual needs at the time. In the course of a treatment, it is not unusual for the practitioner to use their thumbs, fingers, palms, elbows or even feet to apply pressure.

The sensations experienced can vary from treatment to treatment, but most patients describe a temporary sense of tenderness or coldness. However, any discomfort should be minimal and short-lived. You can expect a session to last for approximately 30 minutes to an hour. Initially your practitioner may advise you to have weekly appointments. Once your condition improves, you may feel that less frequent appointments may be sufficient to keep your health in balance.

Bear in mind that you don't need to wait until you are actually ill in order to benefit from acupressure. In common with many of the other complementary therapies encountered in this section, acupressure can be used appropriately in a preventative capacity.

how does acupressure work?

Although it does not involve needles, acupressure has much in common with acupuncture, since both therapies seem to stimulate the production of endorphins in the body. As a result, both appear to encourage a sense of well-being and relaxation.

The benefits attributed to acupressure treatment are wide-ranging and include pain relief, supporting the self-regulating mechanism of the body (including efficient working of the immune system) and releasing muscular tension. In addition, acupressure appears to improve the circulation, thus supporting the detoxification processes of the body. The knock-on effect of this is more efficient transportation of oxygen and vital nutrients, by the blood, to tense areas of the body.

This can encourage the body to fight illness more effectively (for instance stimulating the flow of lymphatic fluid can help to support the immune systems in its fight against infection). Other benefits of a more efficient circulation include decreased lethargy and a greater sense of well-being.

Self-treatment

Self-help acupressure can be a useful tool for treating minor, self-limiting problems (for example, the relief of travel sickness with bands that apply pressure to a specific point on the wrist). However, for more well-established problems, you should seek treatment from a trained practitioner.

ayurveda

Ayurvedic medicine originated in India and its neighbouring countries, but this holistic philosophy is becoming increasingly well-received in the West. This is largely due to the pioneering work of famous practitioners and writers such as Deepak Chopra. The result is the translation of some rather esoteric concepts into up-to-date language that makes sense to us in a modern world with all its attendant stresses and pressures.

In order to appreciate the Ayurvedic approach to healing, you need to understand the basic concepts of the three *doshas* that are believed to be present in each of us. The word *dosha* can be loosely translated as 'pattern of vital energy', which, when in optimum balance, helps to support and maintain a state of good health at mental, emotional and physical levels. Any imbalance results in symptoms of ill health.

the first treatment

Your Ayurvedic practitioner will question you in detail about your general state of health, as well as exploring the specific symptoms of ill health that have brought you to the consulting room. They will also examine your tongue, pulse, eyes, nails and skin.

From this information they will form a picture of your situation and establish a treatment plan. Depending on your needs, this may take the form of a medicine of vegetable, herbal or mineral origin, dietary advice, breathing techniques, massage, meditation, relaxation or deep cleansing.

Remember

You do not need to be struggling with the specific symptoms of an illness before seeking help from an Ayurvedic practitioner. It is equally appropriate to consider treatment if you just feel generally under par and want to take some positive action to boost your health.

how does ayurveda work?

In Ayurvedic medicine, each person's state of health is seen as being fundamentally influenced by three basic energy patterns in the body: *vata* (wind), *pitta* (fire) and *kapha* (earth). Everyone possesses all three of these, but when one or two become dominant the individual may become vulnerable to health problems. Too much *vada* can lead to anxiety, insomnia, nervous exhaustion and distraction; *pitta* can lead to irritability and 'burn-out'; while an excess of *kapha* can lead to weight gain, chilliness and a lack of drive, leading to introversion and lack of confidence. The doshas can also be related to physical build. For instance, those who have a predominance of *kapha* may be chunky and gain weight readily, while a dominant *vata* tendency may lead to a slim build with long bones, and those with a dominance of *pitta* may be well-proportioned with a tendency for skin to be fair and freckle easily.

From the perspective of an Ayurvedic practitioner, these three doshas are not static and fixed, but constantly shifting, changing and adapting according to a variety of factors. These include: poor diet, an unusual amount of stress, lack of physical exercise, sleep deprivation, accumulation of toxins in the system, trauma, surgery or recovery from an accident, and bereavement.

As an example, someone may be born with a dominance of *kapha* in their constitution, but this can be positively modified by taking more gentle exercise (to tone up a sluggish system), eating fewer stodgy foods and resisting the temptation to sleep too much. Like so many other complementary therapies, the Ayurvedic approach to healing is concerned with giving the body the support it needs to achieve an optimum state of balance.

Self-treatment

Assessing what a patient needs to achieve this state of harmony in the system can be tricky, so you need to consult an experienced practitioner in order to get the best chance of a successful outcome.

chinese herbalism

This is one of the major branches of traditional Chinese medicine. Practitioners often prescribe a combination of selected Chinese herbs, often as part of a broader treatment programme that includes acupuncture. The concept of harmony and balance is at the heart of traditional medical theory, often communicated by the yin-yang symbol. In good health, these two principles should be in balance, with neither dominating the other.

The aim is to identify the nature of the imbalance in the system that is leaving the patient vulnerable to ill health. One of the fundamental concepts, common to both acupuncture and Chinese herbalism, is the need for balance and harmony, not only within the body, but also with the environment.

the first treatment

Before making a diagnosis or issuing any prescription, your Chinese herbalist will ask for a wealth of information. While focusing on the problems and symptoms that have made you seek treatment, they will broaden the picture by investigating any lifestyle factors that may have left you vulnerable to symptoms of illness. These include lack of exercise, poor diet, punishing working hours, excessive levels of stress or loss of a partner.

A pattern of head-to-toe questioning enables the herbalist to focus on the main areas of your body that are subject to imbalance. They will often pay special attention to the health of the digestive organs and kidneys, as well as considering patterns of thirst and regularity of bowel movements. In addition, they will take detailed pulse readings, as well as examining the tongue, paying particular attention to its shape, colour and texture. Any coating, discoloration or cracking of the surface may indicate an imbalance elsewhere in the system.

Using this information, the herbalist will draw up a prescription for herbs individually tailored to your specific needs. These come in a variety of forms, such as pills, powders, tinctures or decoctions. Decoctions involve putting a mixture of dried herbs in a saucepan of water and simmering them for about 30 minutes.

how does Chinese herbalism work?

A Chinese herbalist views symptoms of illness in a subtly different light to a conventional Western doctor. For a Western doctor, symptoms (backed up by relevant tests) are a guide to the diagnosis of a specific illness or condition. For a traditional Chinese herbalist, symptoms are an indication of a fundamental state of imbalance or disharmony in the system as a whole. As a result, whatever herbs are prescribed will be aimed at helping the body to rectify this fundamental imbalance and restore a state of harmony.

eczema and Chinese herbalism

There have been many studies on the use of herbal treatment in China, but a study in the United Kingdom of children with eczema at the Hospital for Sick Children in London, showed particularly impressive results. According to the *British Journal of Dermatology*, there was a 60 per cent improvement in response to Chinese herbal treatment and no adverse side-effects.

Self-treatment

Although some Chinese herbs are available over the counter, for long-standing or severe conditions it is advisable to consult an experienced herbalist. Self-treatment with inappropriate herbs may cause problems, especially if you are already taking conventional drugs, which may react with Chinese herbs. To avoid this, always tell your Chinese herbalist about any conventional drugs you have been prescribed. Likewise tell you doctor about any Chinese herbs that you are taking.

shiatsu

The practice of Shiatsu has much in common with acupressure and acupuncture in that all seek to harmonize the flow of chi (vital energy) throughout the whole body. The practitioner uses different types of pressure and stretches with the aim of stimulating the flow of chi along the invisible pathways or meridians, that are believed to exist across the surface of the body. These are the same meridians used in acupuncture and acupressure.

Originating in Japan, shiatsu is becoming increasingly popular in the West as an effective treatment for a range of ailments, as well as for preventive treatment. Shiatsu can help relieve specifically physical problems such as limited mobility, stiffness and pain in joints, as well as promoting a general sense of well-being and relaxation.

the first treatment

Your practitioner will begin by taking a full case history in order to make a clinical evaluation and diagnosis. This will include details of any past treatments and medication. They will also give you a physical examination, taking your pulse, observing your complexion, general health and tone of the skin, looking at your tongue, and palpating the affected areas in order to assess range of movement and strength.

If your practitioner decides that Shiatsu will benefit your problem, treatment can begin. A session usually lasts for about 30–60 minutes and you remain fully clothed. It is therefore important to wear comfortable, loose-fitting clothes. Otherwise, there is no need to make any special preparation apart from avoiding eating a large meal or drinking alcohol.

During the session, you lie on a firm surface, such as a futon, while your practitioner applies graduated pressure to the areas of your body needing attention. As with acupressure, do not be surprised if your practitioner uses their hands, elbows, knees or feet in the course of the treatment.

The intensity of stimulation can vary from very firm to light, depending on what is necessary. Your practitioner may also suggest energizing exercises to support the balanced or enhanced flow of chi through the body.

The movements that the practitioner uses during the treatment may include rubbing and kneading, or maintaining a controlled amount of pressure at one spot. Practitioners often make balanced and controlled use of their body weight, regardless of whether the client is lying on their back, front or sides, or sitting upright. However, this at no time causes a patient undue strain or discomfort.

how does shiatsu work?

The main aim of Shiatsu is to regulate, balance or stimulate the flow of chi throughout the body, by applying pressure or massage to specific points on the body. General benefits are thought to include regulation of the circulatory and lymphatic systems, the increased efficiency of toxin elimination, enhanced hormonal balance, release of muscle tension and deep relaxation.

manipulative therapies

massage

Massage is one of the most pleasurable, comforting and profoundly relaxing forms of treatment available. Helpful for a wide range of stress-related problems, from tension headaches to back and neck and shoulder pain, massage is a hands-on way of encouraging the body to relax. As a result it can help reduce pain that is linked to muscles and joints being held in a tight, tense manner. It can also be of particular benefit to anyone who knows they hold their emotions at bay by tensing their muscles whether they want to or not.

While the immediate benefits of massage are obvious, it is interesting to note that some minor studies have confirmed its psychological benefits. For example, a study in the mid-1990s showed that cardiac patients who were given aromatherapy massage (whether with aromatherapy essential oils or plain carrier oils) showed significant psychological benefits compared with others who received no massage. Another study carried out on institutionalized elderly patients who were given regular back massage confirmed this.

the first treatment

Your therapist will begin by taking a simple case history in order to establish where the problem areas lie and whether you are taking any conventional medicines that might have a bearing on the treatment or suffering from any conditions that might make massage treatment inadvisable.

The therapist will then ask you to remove your clothing while he or she temporarily leaves the room. Since the object of the treatment is for your therapist's hands to make smooth contact with your body, it is helpful to remove as much clothing as you feel at ease with. It is also best to remove any jewellery, such as earrings or necklaces, that might make the treatment uncomfortable when you are lying down.

During the course of the treatment (which can last 60–90 minutes), the therapist will cover your body with a towel and/or blanket to ensure that you do not get cold during the session. This also allows for physical contact while maintaining your modesty. The treatment room should be professionally laid out and maintained, and comfortably warm. This is important because the muscles tend to contract in chilly surroundings, which makes it much more difficult to relax them. Most therapists use a special massage table, sometimes with an oval aperture at one end. This allows you to rest your face in the oval while lying on your stomach, and thus keep your neck straight.

Your therapist will probably use an oil to enhance the flowing movements of their hands over your body. Some therapists suggest using scented aromatherapy essential oils to enhance the relaxing or energizing effect of the treatment.

how does massage work?

In common with other forms of holistic healing that seek to treat and balance the body, massage therapy is thought to support the body's self-healing mechanism. It is particularly helpful in the relief of stress-related problems, partly because of the positive effect it is thought to have on the autonomic nervous system. This system controls the involuntary functioning of the heart, glands and smooth muscles, and regulates the digestion and circulation. Massage also stimulates the circulatory and lymphatic systems, so that waste products are dealt with more efficiently. This can help regulate a sluggish metabolism and help boost and re-balance energy levels. The release of feel-good hormones such as serotonin is also thought to be a benefit of massage treatment.

Self-treatment

If you are following a course of homoeopathic treatment, it may be best if your therapist uses an unscented carrier oil. This is because some aromatherapy oils are thought to interfere with the action of homoeopathic remedies.

osteopathy and cranial osteopathy

Osteopathy involves the use of manipulation in order to obtain the optimum alignment of the musculo-skeletal system. It is an ideal treatment for any condition arising from a mechanical disturbance of the spine and is especially helpful to anyone suffering from stiffness, chronic or acute back pain, postural problems, headaches resulting from tension and stiffness in the neck, or immobility or discomfort resulting from sports injuries. The ultimate aim of osteopathic treatment is to relieve muscle tension, optimize bone and muscle function and, by restoring its self-balancing systems, give the body the best opportunity to heal itself.

Cranial osteopathy is a more recent off-shoot of osteopathy and was developed by an American osteopath Dr William Garner in the 1930s. According to the basic theory of cranial osteopathy, the bones that make up the portion of our skulls known as the cranium retain some degree of flexibility beyond babyhood. It focuses on the need for cerebrospinal fluid (which protects and nourishes the membranes surrounding the brain and spinal cord) to flow in a smooth, rhythmical way. If examinations reveal any disturbance in the flow of this fluid, the cranial osteopath will treat it by very gently manipulating the bones of the cranium and spine.

the first treatment

Your osteopath will take a full case history, questioning you about your current problems, how long you have had them and your state of health. The osteopath will then give you a thorough physical examination, paying particular attention to areas of stiffness, weakness or tenderness, and will probably ask you to perform a simple series of movements in order to assess your flexibility and general range of mobility. On the basis of this information, the osteopath will then form a diagnosis and decide upon a treatment plan.

Treatment usually involves gentle stretching of muscles, rhythmic passive movements of joints or massage of soft tissue. Cranial osteopaths use their finely tuned sense of touch to locate and correct limitations of tissue mobility around the head and neck area, which is believed to have a beneficial effect on the whole body. Any cracking sounds you may hear are caused by air being displaced, not the crunching of bones. Although the crunching or cracking sounds that accompany an osteopathic treatment can be somewhat dramatic this really shouldn't be painful at all.

how does osteopathy work?

Osteopaths believe that many conditions result directly or indirectly from mechanical disturbances of the spine. Establishing the optimum alignment of the spine through manipulation restores the natural balance of the musculo-skeletal system, so that the muscles and bones can move freely. This also gives the internal organs more room to function properly and improves the circulation.

Osteopaths generally acknowledge the links that exist between problems in the skeletal and muscular structure and problems with the balanced functioning of specific organs. As a result, neck pain or tension can be linked to chronic headaches, while poor circulatory function can trigger states of low energy or chronic fatigue.

Cranial osteopathy appears to play a particularly positive role in preventing recurrent ear infections in children. A recent study in the United States revealed that the gentle manipulation encourages fluids to drain more effectively from the head and neck, so that bacteria have nowhere to thrive.

Research into osteopathy

Research into osteopathy has been quite extensive in the United States but there has been criticism of early trials. Since the state registration of osteopaths, more studies have been conducted in the United Kingdom, of which the Department of Health s pilot assessments of the value of osteopathy and chiropractic to the National Health Service are a good example. Results so far suggest that the patients most likely to benefit are those suffering from acute back pain.

chiropractic

Like osteopathy, chiropractic is a 'hands-on' therapy that emerged from the United States. Developed by Daniel D. Palmer in 1895, it is based on the belief that ill health arises if there is abnormal movement in any given joint. Much of a chiropractor's work concentrates on the alignment of the spine, since Palmer was convinced that misaligned (or subluxed) vertebrae or joints was at the centre of an astonishing 95 per cent of most illnesses. Gently restoring the misaligned vertebra to its optimum position can play an invaluable role in maintaining the health of the nervous system, thus allowing good health to re-establish itself.

An impressive amount of scientific research supports the premise that chiropractic treatment can play an extremely positive role in relieving the misery of lower back pain. Results are encouraging from the points of view of both patient satisfaction and cost-effectiveness. Although conventional doctors were initially very sceptical about the merits and medical pedigree of chiropractic, practitioners in the United Kingdom have been state registered since 1994 and have also gained professional recognition and status in the United States.

the first treatment

Your chiropractor will ask you about any traumas, accidents or injuries you sustained as a child or an adult, as well as taking a basic medical history. They will take into account any lifestyle factors that have a bearing on overall health, such as being overweight or unfit, or having a high stress load to deal with on an extended or regular basis. Observation and a physical examination are part of this.

The chiropractor will use this information to identify the source of the problem which will either be a mechanical cause or an underlying condition relating to a specific organ. After making a satisfactory diagnosis, they will explain their proposed treatment plan.

Before starting treatment, the chiropractor will usually ask you to remove all but your underwear and to put on a treatment gown that opens at the back. This allows them to see and feel what is happening to your spine during the course of treatment. For most of the treatment, you will be lying face down on a treatment table.

The basic approach to treatment is a form of manipulation, involving short, precise, thrusting movements to specific parts of the spine and other joints (such as the hips and neck). Soft tissues may also be a focus of attention, and the chiropractor will apply regulated, sustained pressure to specific areas of the body or massage to relaxed tight, tense muscles. Although rather dramatic in the sounds that can occur during a treatment, a chiropractic session should not cause you distress or pain.

They may also advise you on positive lifestyle changes to improve the overall situation, such as dietary changes, weight loss and/or postural improvements (such as wearing shoes with lower heels or not carrying a heavy bag on one shoulder).

how does chiropractic work?

To the chiropractor, the health and alignment of the spine is of central importance. The spine is not only a key support for the body, enabling you to stay upright, but it also protects the nervous system. As a result, any problems affecting the health and alignment of the spine can produce much broader disturbances than just back pain. These include digestive, respiratory, circulatory and hormonal problems.

Chiropractic and trauma

Chiropractic can also be immensely helpful in encouraging the body to settle back into balance again after an accident such as a fall, minor car crash or any other incident that causes trauma to the body.

reflexology

Reflexology is an increasingly popular form of complementary medicine that has a profound and general relaxing effect, as well as giving the therapist and client a perspective on where areas of imbalance may lie in the body. It seems to be helpful in the treatment of back pain, period problems, asthma, anxiety and multiple sclerosis. It is likely to appeal to anyone who responds well to a direct, hands-on approach. Some reflexologists may also be happy to provide additional advice about healthy lifestyle changes that will contribute to improvements in overall health and vitality.

the first treatment

The reflexologist will ask you about your medical history and usually about your overall state of health and lifestyle. Once you have removed your footwear, they will then examine your feet. During treatment your feet will be raised so that the reflexologist can work on them effectively. You should feel comfortable at all times. Treatment can sometimes be temporarily painful or pleasurably relaxing, depending on what the reflexologist is aiming to do. Although reflexology is most often understood to involve work with the feet, pressure points on the hand can also be used during a treatment.

During a treatment, the reflexologist moves their thumb and fingers slowly over the surface of the sole, using small, precise movements. This allows them to identify any tender or sensitive areas. These are the points that can indicate where underlying problems lurk in the body. The aim of applying pressure in this precise way is to break up tiny, crystal-like deposits in the feet. It is also believed to improve circulation, release blockages in energy flow and allow a freer passage of nerve impulses.

During the course of a treatment your reflexologist will note any areas of your feet that seem tender or sensitive. Developing calluses or skin eruptions such as eczema, may be a sign of poor blood supply.

A treatment lasts for approximately 60 minutes and your reflexologist will advise you about the number of visits you will need. This could be once a week, or even two or three times a week initially if your problems need particular attention. Once the problems have cleared up, you may decide to continue having the occasional treatment in order to provide some sort of health check.

how does reflexology work?

In reflexology the feet are regarded as a mirror image of the body, the right foot representing the right side of the body and the left foot representing the left side. There is thought to be a connection between specific areas of the feet and particular organs or parts of the body, so that applying pressure to a specific point on the foot also affects the corresponding organ. Reflexology is also thought to have a potentially beneficial effect on the whole body by releasing stress and tension, stimulating the self-healing mechanism of the body and generally inducing a sense of well-being and vitality.

Reflexology and Zone Therapy

Reflexology owes a huge debt to an American physician Dr William Fitzgerald, who worked in the early twentieth century. Fitzgerald developed a system of treatment called Zone Therapy that involved applying pressure to specific parts of the body in order to achieve a pain-relieving effect elsewhere. According to Zone Therapy, the body consists of ten zones, made up of vertical sections that run from the toes to the top of the head and down again to the hands. These zones are thought to be linked by energy flow (rather like the meridian theory of traditional Chinese medicine). As a result, controlled pressure on one part of the body can affect another part of the body in the same zone.

natural therapies

aromatherapy

Aromatherapy is becoming increasingly popular because of the pleasurable nature of using essential oils in massage blends, inhalation or bath products. Because of its practical nature, aromatherapy has none of the mystique of the more esoteric therapies, such as Ayurveda and homoeopathy. Therefore it is ideally suited to self-treatment. Because of its holistic nature, aromatherapy aims to treat the whole body, encouraging mind, emotions and physical health to reach an optimum state of balance.

Recent research studies appear to support some of the therapeutic claims for aromatherapy (such as the role of specific essential oils in inducing a state of relaxation and improved sleep). In the mid-1990s, one study, praised for its sound design, examined the effects of selected essential oils on smooth muscle, found in areas like the bladder and stomach which are not under conscious control and on 25 species of bacteria and 3 species of fungi. The results confirmed that essential oils of geranium, neroli, patchouli, peppermint, lavender and marjoram had a relaxing effect on smooth muscle. Conversely, essential oils of bergamot, clary sage, lemon grass, fennel, frankincense, lemon and rosemary produced muscle spasms.

Tea tree oil proved active against 24 of the 25 strains of bacteria tested, as well as having impressive anti-fungal properties. Other essential oils that help fight bacteria include bergamot, lavender, marjoram, neroli, thyme and rosemary.

the first treatment

Your aromatherapist should be well versed in the medicinal uses of essential oils, as well as having a basic understanding of the anatomy and physiology of the body. A knowledge of physiology is particularly relevant to the use of essential oils for massage.

After taking a brief case history, your aromatherapist will produce a blend of the essential oils most likely to benefit your current situation. These oils can be used in a variety of ways, the most popular being direct application to the skin in the form of a massage blend, or inhalation of the aromas produced from an oil-burner.

Your aromatherapist may offer some practical advice about lifestyle changes, such as stress-management techniques, appropriate exercise, and/or improving the balance and quality of your diet.

how does aromatherapy work?

The essential oils used in aromatherapy are highly concentrated substances that contain a range of chemicals, including alcohols, esters, aldehydes and terpenes. It is precisely this complex nature that is believed to endow them with such an impressively broad range of therapeutic properties. As a result, a single essential oil may have antidepressant, analgesic, sedative and/or antiseptic properties.

Because their molecules are so minute, essential oils are thought to enter the bloodstream through contact with the skin, or through the tissues of the lungs through inhalation. Although essential oils are sometimes taken by mouth in parts of mainland Europe, this is not a recommended practice in the United Kingdom. Instead, the most common routes of absorption of any tailor-made blend of oils are massage or inhalation.

Aromatherapy can address a fairly wide range of chronic health conditions, the most common being skin conditions, menstrual problems and stress-related conditions.

Self-treatment

Home use of essential oils is also a practical option. However, before doing so, it is very important to attend an introductory course on the subject in order to ensure that the oils are used in the safest and most effective way.

homeopathy

Homeopathic medicine is an extremely flexible and practical approach to healing that was developed in Germany just over 200 years ago. It was developed by Samuel Hahneman in the early eighteenth century and is based on the principle of 'like treats like'. The medicines are of plant, animal or mineral origin and are used in progressive greater dilutions, or 'potencies', based on either a decimal or centesimal scale. The most dilute remedies have the greatest potency. This is because the shaking at each dilution is thought to energize, or potentiate, the ingredient.

the first treatment

Some patients are astonished to find themselves spending 60–90 minutes talking about their current health problems within the context of their overall medical history. However, seeing how quickly time passes for each new patient once they relax and settle into the consultation is one of the delights of being a homoeopath. In fact, many patients say that the initial consultation itself has therapeutic value.

Your homeopath will start by asking incredibly detailed questions about the problem that has brought you for treatment in the first place, such as the factors that make the symptoms feel better or worse, any obvious triggers to their onset, and the existence or quality of any pain. From this information, they can gain a fairly accurate picture of your psychological, emotional and physical well-being within the time available.

The homeopath has then to make sense of all this information by carrying out a case analysis. To do this, they will consult reference books or, increasingly, avail themselves tailor-made computer software for case analysis. Once the analysis is complete, they will be in a position to select the homoeopathic remedy that is most appropriate for your overall combination of symptoms.

The remedy may take the form of a single tablet or a course of tablets to be taken daily for a specified period of time. Alternatively it may be in the form of a liquids, powder, globule (a round pill) or granules.

how does homeopathy work?

Because it involves the use of extraordinarily dilute medicines, controversy has raged over how this gentle, holistic form of medicine can work. Conventional doctors frequently attribute any benefits to the placebo effect (or 'mind over matter') but the question remains open. A number of tentative theories have been (and are still being) put forward. One suggests that the molecules of the water used in the process of extreme dilution act as a template, taking on board an imprint or 'memory' of the active ingredient.

Unlike conventional drugs, which are usually aimed at suppressing the symptoms of a disorder, homoeopathic medicines mimic the symptoms in the belief that they are part of the disorder and should be allowed to run their full course. In this way, they gently but effectively stimulate the body's own self-healing mechanism. Occasionally a patient may feel worse before they get better.

Homeopathic remedies – some basic rules

If you opt for self-treatment, be guided by the following:

• Look for the remedy that provides the closest match to your symptoms.

• Take only one remedy at a time.

• The most appropriate self-help dose is 6c (this refers to a centesimal scale of dilution based on 1 part/drop of the remedy to 99 parts of the dilutant). These should be available from most high-street pharmacies and health-food shops or in some supermarkets. For problems of recent onset, take one dose hourly for up to 3 hours. For more slow-developing, low-grade symptoms, take one dose 3 times a day for a maximum of 3 days.

• Once symptoms improve, stop taking the remedy, because this is a sign that the body is beginning to cope by itself. If you do not see any improvement after taking 3 doses a day for a maximum of 3 days, you should look for another remedy or another solution.

nutritional approaches

Most people are familiar with the phrase: 'We are what we eat'. Trite as it sounds, this contains a basic truth: the food that we eat every day not only provides the basic materials for our bodies to build, renew and repair our cells but also provides the fuel that drives the body's activities and keeps us warm. With this in mind, it is easy to appreciate that a consistently low-quality diet will probably result in a mediocre state of health, with reduced vitality and a vulnerability to infections.

Most research into nutritional therapy concerns the effectiveness of exclusion diets in patients with a range of chronic health problems. Such diets involve the exclusion from the diet, for a specific time, of any foods suspected of aggravating the symptoms of illness. If this produces signs of general improvement, individual foods are gradually re-introduced to see whether symptoms re-appear.

Scientific trials indicate that conditions such as rheumatoid arthritis, irritable bowel syndrome, candida, hyperactivity in children, migraine, asthma and eczema all respond positively to exclusion diets.

the first treatment

Your nutritional therapist will take a detailed case history, considering your current health problems within the context of your overall medical history. The initial consultation will last for about an hour, which gives them enough time to assess your general level of health and to take into consideration any conventional drugs that you are currently being prescribed

On the basis of this information, they may suggest some tests, such as analyzing blood samples for food intolerances or hair for minerals.

Whatever the therapist's advice, it should take into account your individual constitution and personality. This applies not only to dietary changes or nutritional supplements but also to lifestyle changes that may contribute to overall health.

It will also be helpful to be frank with your nutritional therapist about how to achieve and maintain sensible and realistic changes in your diet. Should you feel some suggestions are too hard or radical, this needs to be honestly discussed.

how does nutritional therapy work?

Specific nutritional deficiencies will obviously respond to nutritional supplements (for instance, vitamin B12 for pernicious anaemia and vitamin B1 for beri beri). However, in the Western world, many people, despite being overweight, are still suffering from low-grade malnutrition because their diet lacks essential nutrients. This situation is further complicated by the vast array of chemical additives in our foods, such as preservatives, flavourings and colourings.

To overcome low-grade malnutrition of this kind requires the re-introduction of basic nutritional elements into the diet. The advice of any nutritional therapist is likely to include:

• The addition of certain foods to the diet.

• Healthier forms of food preparation (such as steaming, which preserves the vitamin content).

• Regular meals.

• Vitamin and/or mineral supplements.

• The use of fresh organic foods rather than frozen or tinned foods.

In addition, it is also the job of the nutritional therapist to give advice on what to limit or avoid, such as:

• Anti-nutrients (such as heavy metals, antibiotics, artificial hormones or alcohol).

• Low-grade dehydration.

• Foods that may be triggering negative symptoms.

naturopathy

This holistic system of healing aims to strengthen the body's capacity to maintain good health and effectively fight off disease. One of the central tenets of naturopathy is the belief that many illnesses are caused by a build-up of toxic wastes in the body. As a result, learning how to gently but effectively encourage the body to detox is a central concern of naturopathic treatments. This may take the form of dietary modifications, hydrotherapy techniques, or the use of herbal or homeopathic medicines.

In common with homoeopathy, the naturopathic approach is not about suppressing the symptoms of ill health. Instead it aims to:

• Identify the source of the problem.

• Rectify any imbalance in the system.

• Administer whatever combination of complementary treatments is necessary to support the body's attempts to throw off illness.

Using a combination of different complementary approaches to healing, a naturopath aims to strengthen the patient's entire system on mental, emotional and physical levels. This is important, since from the naturopathic point of view, illness affects the whole body, so that treatment seldom targets any specific organ in isolation.

the first treatment

This usually lasts for about an hour, during which your naturopath will examine all aspects of your health. They will ask detailed questions about your medical history, postural and working habits, eating patterns and diet, regularity of bowel movements, general levels of vitality and well-being, and the overall stress levels that you experience on a daily basis.

They will also carry out a number of routine tests, such as measuring your blood pressure and assessing your lung function, range of movement of joints, muscle strength and body reflexes. They may also take blood and/or urine samples for analysis, as well as examining the iris of your eye for diagnostic purposes, or to establish whether you show any signs of mineral imbalance or toxic metal accumulation.

Using this information, your naturopath will tailor a treatment plan to meet your specific health needs. This may involve:

• Referral to your doctor for further tests.

• Dietary changes.

• Strictly regulated periods of fasting.

• Hydrotherapy.

• Relaxation techniques.

In addition, your naturopath may offer acupuncture, soft-tissue massage, osteopathy, herbal remedies or homoeopathic treatment as a gentle way of supporting your body towards a better state of health.

Treatment should result in a steady and cumulative improvement in the quality of your overall health, possibly punctuated by occasional short-lived relapses or 'healing crises'. Some symptoms may re-appear briefly (often in the reverse order of their initial emergence) or progress from internal parts of the body to more superficial, external levels. For instance, if you have a digestive or respiratory problem, this will probably clear up before a skin condition such as eczema or psoriasis.

how does naturopathy work?

Naturopathic treatments are aimed at supporting and stimulating the self-healing, self-regulating and self-balancing potential of the body rather than subduing and suppressing the symptoms of illness. As a result, naturopaths regard health as a positive experience rather than just a state in which no symptoms of illness are evident.

A naturopath may suggest any of the following measures.

• Nutritional improvements – an increased intake of fresh fruit and vegetables (through juicing) and of raw and/or unprocessed foods, and possibly controlled fasting. Naturopaths believe that these dietary measures enable the body to detoxify more efficiently.

• Soft-tissue massage and/or osteopathy combined with hydrotherapy – to benefit physical health by promoting optimum alignment of the spine and relaxing the muscles. They can positively benefit stress-related conditions.

• Counselling and stress-management techniques – as a means of relieving the feelings of distress that sometimes accompany chronic illness, especially if it brings pain in its wake.

western herbalism

This is one of the best-established, most accessible branches of complementary medicine and has an impressive track record in providing effective, natural medicines that seem to act more gently than their conventional counterparts. This appears to be partly due to the way that herbalists make use of the whole plant rather than a highly concentrated extract (as favoured by the conventional pharmaceutical industry).

This particular branch of herbal medicine (or phytotherapy as it is sometimes called) occurs in the West, but it is important to be aware that some form of herbal medicine occurs world-wide. According to the World Health Organization, the use of herbal medicine on a global basis outweighs that of conventional medicine by three to four times. This is partly due to the fact that, in many parts of the world, people do not have access to conventional medicine. Herbalism was also widely practised in the West until about 200 years ago, largely because the only alternative was an untrained, expensive 'doctor'. As a legacy of these times, many conventional drugs in general use are derived from traditional herbal remedies.

the first treatment

Your herbalist will begin by gathering enough information to put together a detailed case history. They will question you about the health of the major systems of your body (such as the digestive and respiratory systems), take blood pressure readings and possibly examine the iris of your eye.

On the basis of this information, the herbalist will then prescribe whatever herbal formula is most appropriate. Medicines take the form of tinctures, capsules, tablets, teas, creams, ointments or essential plant oils.

Research on St John's wort

One of the most impressive and persuasive series of scientific trials involved the use of St John's Wort in the treatment of mild to moderate depression. In 1996, the British Medical Journal published a systematic review of 23 clinical trials of this herbal treatment. Patients given St John's Wort were two and a half times more likely to respond favourably than those given a placebo. Comparisons of treatments with St John's Wort and conventional antidepressants showed a favourable response in 20 per cent of patients treated with St John's Wort. There are questions over the advisability of taking St John's Wort with some conventional medicines, so always check with your pharmacist or doctor before considering it.

how does western herbalism work?

The Western herbalism approach has a great deal in common with other major systems of complementary therapy, such as traditional Chinese medicine and homoeopathy. All are based on the concept that the body has a self-regulating, self-healing mechanism that functions harmoniously in good health but falls into a state of imbalance in times of illness.

Western herbalism aims to restore the balance and equilibrium of the whole body rather than temporarily suppressing symptoms of ill health. Therefore, any herbal preparations prescribed may produce a range of protective reactions from the body, such as:

• Detoxifying the system.

• Supporting the circulatory system.

• Soothing calm irritated and/or inflamed skin and mucus membranes.

Because herbal preparations involve the use of whole plants, rather than just their active ingredients, their effects are thought to be synergistic. This means that the action of the active ingredient is enhanced or modified, so that it has a gentler, but still very positive effect on the body. This contrasts markedly with conventional medicines, which are a concentration of active ingredients that are more likely to produce side-effects.

bach flower remedies

The profile of these immensely popular and easy-to-use remedies has received a huge boost from the attention given to the Rescue Remedy formula by the popular press. This is a non-addictive, gentle formula for the treatment of symptoms arising from minor accidents, stress or trauma and its success is hardly surprising. Bach flower remedies are gentle, non-addictive liquid medicines that can be used to help ease a number of mild to moderate emotional problems. The medicines are made by exposing plants and water to sunlight, or using a boiling technique to produce a mother tincture.

Although they have only become generally available in the last few years, the 38 flower remedies date back to the work of Dr Edward Bach in the 1930s. A conventional doctor by training, Bach became convinced that there must be a more effective and humane way of gently restoring the body, mind and emotions to good health other than by using conventional drugs. Thinking along these lines, he became interested in the work of another conventionally trained doctor who had become similarly disillusioned with his work: Samuel Hahnemann, the founder of homoeopathy.

In his early medical work, Bach began to feel that, although he was treating their physical ailments, he was not helping his patients to address the deeper emotional issues and conflicts that were undermining their overall health.

In 1928, with this in mind, Bach spent some time in Wales where he began to work along purely intuitive lines, exploring preparations of wild flowers such as Impatiens, Mimulus and Clematis. According to contemporary accounts, Bach used to experience a number of intense physical and psychological symptoms before finding an appropriate flower remedy. He would then go into the countryside, where he would be drawn to the wild flower that would relieve his symptoms.

the first treatment

Practitioners specializing in the use of Bach flower remedies are rare. More often, these remedies are suggested by complementary practitioners working in other fields as an additional avenue of support. For instance, homoeopaths often suggest using Rescue Remedy in combination with an acute homoeopathic remedy for trauma, while reflexologists or naturopaths may suggest a blend of flower essences for support during a difficult, demanding or stressful emotional time.

how do bach flower remedies work?

During his medical career, Bach concluded that ill health results from a persistent imbalance or lack of harmony between the emotional, mental and physical states. As a result, he felt strongly that disease was a result of a persistently negative mindset. We can therefore see his work as an interesting forerunner of the newly emerging scientific field of psycho-neuro-immunology, which examines the powerful link between state of mind, emotions and health.

Bach was very much ahead of his time in his implicit belief in the need to treat the whole person rather than trying to suppress individual symptoms routinely or in isolation. He took an uncompromising perspective on illness, seeing it as the result of a patient losing the ability to tune into their intuition and follow their positive instincts.

As a result, Bach viewed people as becoming vulnerable to the experience and progression of illness, as if a basic resistance blocked the balanced development of their true personality. In his opinion, these blocks took the form of negative emotions, such as anxiety, anger, resentment or intolerance. Therefore, his flower remedies aim to re-establish emotional and mental balance. In this way, they are appropriate for use in emotional crises, although they also have a preventive use.

Self-treatment

Flower remedies are suitable for self-treatment because they are available over the counter and easy to use, given the aid of a reliable reference book. Safe, non-addictive and free of known side-effects, they are a gentle source of complementary medical support for demanding situations. While popular, Bush essences are still fairly new, so keep it simple and stick to Bach.

active therapies

meditation and visualization

The benefits of regular mediation or visualization are wide-ranging and well documented. Studies have shown significant improvements in mental focus and concentration levels in people who regularly practise transcendental meditation. Other positive effects include a lessening of anxiety-related irritability, aggression, mood swings, rapid heartbeat, insomnia and hyperventilation (rapid, shallow breathing). All these effects are related to the 'fight or flight' response of the sympathetic branch of the autonomic nervous system. The secretion of the stress hormones adrenalin and cortisol is an integral part of a typical stress response.

Studies have repeatedly shown that the practice of meditation or visualization helps us to switch on the parasympathetic part of the autonomic nervous system. This allows us to experience positive physiological changes that can be described as the relaxation response. This has the opposite effects of the negative, stress-related symptoms described above, and includes a decrease in oxygen consumption because of relaxed breathing patterns; lowered heart rate, reduced levels of blood lactate – which can cause tense and aching muscles – and a general sense of profound relaxation.

learning how to meditate

If you are taught to meditate and do so daily, you can experience benefits in the form of reduced problems with anxiety, sleep problems, high blood pressure, and any aches and pains related to holding muscles in a state of constant tension. Because your concentration improves, you can also realistically expect to become generally more focused, creative and productive.

Learning to meditate gives you the ability to consciously switch off the distracting 'chatter' that goes through your mind on the average day. Left unattended, these random thoughts can prove a major obstacle to focusing productively on any task in hand.

A simple meditation technique is quite easy to learn. It helps if you dress in loose comfortable clothing and lie on a flat surface or sit in a straight-backed chair that gives maximum support to the spine. Close your eyes and focus on your breathing, regulating it gently so that it becomes slower and more rhythmical. On no account force your breathing to take on any particular pattern or rhythm.

If you prefer to meditate in an upright position with your eyes open, it may help if you focus on an object in front of you, such as a flower, candle flame or crystal. Focus on this object as you regulate your breathing, consciously putting aside any intruding thoughts. As you concentrate on the pattern of your breathing, gently regulate it into a steady pattern, in which the inhalation equals the exhalation. To help you focus, repeat a single syllable to yourself as you breathe in and out. This need be nothing more complicated than repeating the sound 'one' gently to yourself.

You can regard visualization as a mental holiday. Close your eyes and focus on images, sounds and sensations that give you especially good feelings. For example, you could recall an image of a place that you have visited, or you could dream up your own special retreat where you feel safe, comfortable and deeply relaxed.

how do meditation and visualization work?

The common element in both these techniques is the switching off of the 'fight or flight' response of the sympathetic branch of the autonomic nervous system and the switching on of the parasympathetic branch.

Once you become adept at switching on the relaxation response you can use it whenever you begin to feel the pressure build. it can be done on a train while travelling to work, at your desk in a break, or even while you are in a shopping queue.

alexander technique

This system of postural counselling enables us to identify areas of tension and misalignment in the body that may be having a negative effect on overall health. We are all aware that the way we feel affects the way we hold ourselves: for instance, if we feel down, we are likely to hunch our shoulders; if we feel confident and outgoing, we hold up our heads. However, we may be less aware that the postural habits we have built up over a lifetime can have a major impact on our mental and emotional health. This concept is at the heart of the Alexander technique.

Learning the Alexander technique is about identifying the negative postural strategies that we have developed over the years (usually in response to stressful triggers that make us feel threatened in some way). Once we identify them, we can exchange them for more favourable, stress-reducing habits.

the first treatment

Before making a physical assessment, the Alexander teacher will require a brief medical history. For part of this, they may ask you to sit on and get out of a chair while they observe the way in which you hold yourself during this simple action. For part of the treatment you may have to lie on an examination table. Unlike a massage or osteopathic session, you will probably remain fully clothed throughout but it is best to wear loose-fitting, comfortable, adequately warm clothes.

Your teacher's task is to spot any postural habits that are encouraging you to hold tension in your muscles and joints. This tension is often referred to as 'pulling down', and it can use up a great deal of your unconscious energy, as well as resulting in a great of deal of muscle tension and discomfort in your joints.

The freedom that comes from learning new ways of holding your body, especially when faced with challenging or difficult situations, can be exhilarating. At first, you may find the adoption of better postural habits and the letting go of more negative ones quite a challenge. This is because, at first, you may long to go back to the habits that feel like second nature.

Your Alexander teacher may also give you 'homework' in the form of some simple exercises between sessions. This could be something as simple as lying on your back on the floor with your knees bent and your head resting on a small pile of books.

how does the alexander technique work?

According to the philosophy of the Alexander technique, breaking negative postural habits and introducing new, positive ones is of enormous benefit to overall health and well-being. This is mainly due to the way in which poor postural trends result in muscles and joints being held in a constantly tense and ultimately distorted state. It is these areas of tension that can lead to chronic problems, such as recurrent tension headaches, migraines, back pain, general pain, stiffness and a limited range of movement.

One delightful bonus of regularly practising the Alexander technique is a slowly increasing level of energy and vitality. This is thought to be associated with the amount of energy involved in unconsciously holding the body in a state of tension. Once these areas of tension become relaxed, the energy can be used more productively.

Do expect your body to offer some resistance to taking on these new postural habits since the older, negative ones will feel more familiar. However, once you persist, you will gently adjust to the new way of holding your body. The health benefits that come from this are well worth the effort.

hypnotherapy

Many of us associate hypnotherapy with the treatment of phobias or addiction to smoking, but it has much broader applications. It also plays a role in the relief of health problems such as insomnia, stress-related conditions, migraine, digestive conditions, pain control (including obstetric applications), period problems and skin conditions such as psoriasis and eczema. Don't be misled or put off by the more sensationalist aspects of 'stage' hypnotherapy with its rather dramatic presentation. This is by no means all there is to this therapy.

The British Society for Experimental and Clinical Hypnosis has compiled a databank from studies of hypnotherapy. Since hypnotherapy does not lend itself to standard double-blind clinical trials, most studies compare the response to hypnotherapy with that of other forms of treatment.

Studies conducted in the late 1980s in the UK on people with asthma have shown marked improvement after hypnotherapy. In one study, patients receiving a 6-week course of hypnotherapy were able to reduce their bronchodilator (inhaler) medication by an overall 26 per cent. In another study of 16 patients with chronic asthma who were given hypnotherapy treatment, hospital admissions in the following year dropped from an average of 44 to an impressive 13.

the first treatment

Your hypnotherapist will take a case history along with relevant details of your current health problems. They will probably also test your susceptibility to hypnosis by inducing a light hypnotic state. To do this, they speak in a relaxing, slow and confident way and you should remain conscious throughout the exercise. They may use images, scene-setting, colour or repeated key statements. Alternatively, they may induce visual concentration by asking you to focus on an object, such as a light, pencil or pendulum.

As you move deeper into a relaxed state, they may suggest that your eyes are getting heavy and want to gently close. However, this does not mean that you will be in a heavy trance state, and you will still be aware of your surroundings and of any suggestions made by your hypnotherapist.

The hypnotherapist is also likely to teach you how to induce a state of relaxation yourself, through auto-hypnosis. Listening to cassette tapes or CDs, which your therapist will recommend, may help you to do this.

how does hypnotherapy work?

Over several sessions a hypnotherapist may take patients into a deeper state of relaxation, where they can safely re-experience old, unresolved conflicts, anxieties or distressing circumstances buried in the subsconscious mind. An experienced hypnotherapist can bring these to the surface at the appropriate time. By doing so, hypnotherapy is thought to allow us to identify and resolve inner conflicts that we may have been unconsciously carrying around since childhood. As a result, we may find an improvement not only in our emotional states, such as relief from anxiety and panic attacks, but also in physical symptoms suspected to be stress-related. These can include a stress-related eczema, asthma, irritable bowel syndrome or recurrent tension headaches and/or migraines.

autogenic training and biofeedback

Autogenic training is a system of deep relaxation developed by a European neurologist Dr Schultz. The training involves focusing the mind on a specific set of mental exercises that should be performed each day in order to gain maximum benefit. As with other forms of deep relaxation, regularity of practice is essential in order to fully benefit from the technique. As a result, it is very helpful to build a short period of time into each day when you can do these exercises undisturbed.

Once you have learned the basic exercises with the help of an experienced practitioner, you can use them to induce a deeply relaxed state within a relatively short period of time.

The use of biofeedback dates back to the 1960s, when scientists working with patients suffering from high blood pressure discovered that biofeedback devices could be used to control and reduce stress-related symptoms. The aim of biofeedback is to teach patients how to gain conscious control over symptoms of stress, such as muscle tension, hyperventilation, neck and shoulder pain, and tension headaches.

the first treatment

After taking a medical history, the practitioner will teach you the six basic exercises (which take the form of specific suggestions) that are at the heart of autogenic training. Each suggestion focuses the mind on actively experiencing a series of sensations in specific parts of the body. This usually takes the form of repeating a direct suggestion to yourself, such as 'my arm is getting heavy' or 'my hand is feeling warm.' At the same time, attention is focused on breathing patterns and heart rhythm.

Generally speaking, it is better to learn the skills of autogenic training from an experienced practitioner than trying to teach yourself at home. In this way you can be sure that you are carrying out the instructions correctly. Also the professional support of an experienced practitioner is invaluable should any unexpected psychological reactions surface. Although this is uncommon, it is immensely helpful to have a practitioner on hand to offer help and advice about how best to proceed.

During a biofeedback session, you are linked by electrodes and probes to a feedback machine. As the session progresses, a series of beeps, flashes or moving needles on the biofeedback device reveals any changes that are happening in your body, such as a decrease or increase in heart rate or a tensing or relaxing of muscles.

Variations in skin temperature, perspiration levels, brain-wave activity, heart rate and muscle tension are all ways of establishing how stressed or relaxed we are. For example, a deeply relaxed state is associated with little perspiration, a slow, steady heart rate and high levels of alpha waves. Therefore, any objective measurements of these signs and symptoms are an indication of just how under pressure we are feeling at any given moment.

The ultimate objective of biofeedback is to make you aware of when certain techniques, such as muscle relaxation and calming breathing strategies, are inducing a state of conscious relaxation. Its beauty is that it can demonstrate in terms of objective responses that relaxation measures are working. This can give us the confidence to use these pro-active, stress-reducing measures whenever necessary.

As a result we can have some positive control over reducing unpleasant stress-related symptoms, such as anxiety and muscular aches and pains. Tension headaches, migraines, high blood pressure, irritable bowel syndrome and insomnia all respond especially well to biofeedback.

how do autogenic training and biofeedback work?

Autogenic training and biofeedback both have a great deal in common with other systems, such as visualization and meditation, that allow us to switch on the relaxation response. In all cases, we are encouraging the parasympathetic branch of the autonomic nervous system to kick in. Once this happens, we feel noticeably calmer, focused and more in control.

yoga

Although yoga has recently experienced a huge surge in popularity, it is no newcomer to the health and fitness scene. In fact it is one of the oldest systems of movement and has a well-established reputation for the promotion of harmony of body and mind. The benefits of yoga are almost too numerous to mention, but the balancing of energy levels is a good place to start. Depending on our needs at any given time, the practice of yoga can help us to be revitalized and more relaxed.

The umbrella term 'yoga' covers several different forms of this system of movement, and what you choose depends on your taste, temperament and level of fitness. Forms of yoga include:

Hatha yoga for generally toning up the muscles, increasing or developing flexibility and learning revitalizing or relaxing breathing techniques. This is a good form of yoga for the beginner.

Iyengar yoga which uses the same basic system of movement but requires greater precision, accuracy and physical strength in order to hold the postures long enough to derive the greatest benefit.

Astanga or 'power' yoga which is a fast-moving system of yoga suitable for anyone who is already very physically fit, toned and coordinated, and who enjoys a challenge. Regular practice should promote a leaner, stronger, more supple physique.

Attending a yoga class on a regular basis will help to build up physical stamina, muscle strength and flexibility, while encouraging the use of breathing techniques to maximize the benefits of the postures. Yoga can also have profound benefit on the mind and emotions, such as switching on the relaxation response and helping the mind to focus. Some postures are thought to lift a low mood or calm the nervous system.

Choosing a form of yoga

Whatever form of yoga you are considering, always check with the teacher in advance. Questions to ask include:

• Is it suited to your general fitness level?

• Do the exercises take into account any severe medical conditions, or any prescription medication that could make you dizzy or uncoordinated?

This does not necessarily mean that yoga is not for you, just that particular postures may need to be adapted or omitted.

the first session

Whatever form of yoga you choose, it is good to remember that it can be adapted to suit your needs and capabilities as your fitness, confidence and general stamina grow.

When learning any system of yoga, do not be tempted to take a short cut and rely on a videotape or DVD. These are a great back-up once you have fully mastered the poses in a class, especially if you like to exercise at home. However, to get the maximum benefit from yoga postures, it is essential to do them correctly. This can only be learned in a small class with an experienced teacher or on a one-to-one basis.

Always choose clothes that are comfortable, non-restrictive and warm enough when doing a yoga class. You don't want to be distracted by feeling restricted or too cold when relaxing at the end of a class.

At the end of any yoga session, there should always be an extended period of relaxation to let your mind and body release any tension. During this time, you are likely to be taught how to breathe in a full and relaxed way, using your diaphragm (the sheet of muscle at the base of the lungs and the rib cage). Learning how to do this is invaluable, since it is one of the most effective stress-releasing tools at our disposal.

how does yoga work?

The regular practice of yoga with its stretching, twisting, turning and holding postures combined with controlled breathing appears to stimulate the nerves and internal organs while soothing the nervous system. The deep breathing techniques taught in yoga class also appear to stimulate blood supply to the internal organs, which is claimed to have a generally revitalizing and rejuvenating effect. When breathing techniques are combined with the controlled movements of the postures, it is said that this can have a de-toxifying effect on the liver, kidneys and spleen.

tai chi

Tai chi was originally developed over 1000 years ago as a martial art in China. Although there are a number of form and variations, the system we may be most familiar with is called the Short Yang Form. This was developed by Cheng Man Ch'ing who lived from 1900 to 1975. Credited as being a renowned teacher of tai chi, Cheng Man Ch'ing was also trained in the use of herbal medicines, as well as having an artistic side that found expression through literature, painting and calligraphy.

The Short Yang Form was developed with the aim of communicating the principles of tai chi to a Western audience, while also promoting the concept of the multiple health-enhancing potential of this gentle, graceful system of movement. In the West it has acquired a powerful reputation as a system of exercise best described as 'meditation in movement'. Much more than merely a way of encouraging the body to become fitter, more coordinated and balanced, tai chi appears to have a huge potential for improving our experience of overall health and well-being at several levels at once. These benefits are said to include more balance energy levels, increased harmony of mind, emotions and body, a profound sense of tranquillity, improved confidence and greater muscle tone.

the first session

At a class you will be taught a series of flowing movements that are accompanied by regular, consciously controlled breathing techniques. Regular practice of tai chi is thought to encourage a more balanced flow of energy (or chi) through the body, and in this way, has much in common with the approaches of acupuncture and acupressure.

The flowing movements of tai chi appear to enhance this improved flow of energy along the invisible pathways called meridians that are believed to traverse the body. While executing

these movements, attention is focused on the area situated just beneath the navel which is sometimes referred to as the 'vital centre' of the body.

By working with this area and directing many of the slow movements from it, internal energy can be consciously directed to the hands and feet. This may not bring any sensation with it, or it can be felt as a tingling, hot or cool sensation.

Regularity of practice is thought to be essentially important in order to make progress and enjoy maximum benefit from this re-balancing system of movement. The best times are thought to be early in the morning or in the evening, ideally aiming for a daily practice session. Attending a class is definitely to be recommended in order to make sure you are executing the movements as correctly as possible. This work can be backed up with regular home practice, if possible in the fresh, open air close to a green space and/or the sound of running water.

how does tai chi work?

The physical benefits claimed for tai chi include greater range of movement in the joints and muscles, better muscle tone and strength, and enhanced postural alignment. In addition, and perhaps, most significantly, tai chi teaches us how to coordinate our breathing with the flowing movements, which makes us more relaxed and energized, while also improving overall balance and physical coordination.

The breathing techniques associated with tai chi can be of particular help to those of us with a tendency to hyperventilate (breathing quickly and shallowly from the upper chest) whenever we feel tense and anxious. Learning how to breathe in a gentle, relaxed way can be the key factor to replacing negative breathing patterns with more positive, tranquil ones. As a result, tai chi can be a hugely effective system of movement in de-stressing mind, emotions and body.

Positive effects of tai chi on fighting illness

Apart from all of the health benefits listed above, tai chi can also play an important role in supporting immune system functioning through stimulating the effective flow of lymphatic fluid. Because the movement of lymphatic fluid is dependent on the regular contraction and relaxation of the muscles in the arms and legs to keep it moving, regular practice of tai chi is a perfect system of movement in supporting this process.

pilates

Although the Pilates system of exercise was developed by Joseph Pilates as a form of physiotherapy, it has met with a huge surge of interest in the last two decades or so. Joseph Pilates was born in Dusseldorf in 1880, suffering very poor physical health as a result of asthma, rickets and rheumatic fever. Rather than accepting the unfortunate level of physical fitness he'd been dealt, Pilates met the challenge by throwing himself into a combination of body-conditioning exercises. His body was transformed to the point where he became a gymnast and adept at yoga and the martial arts.

Pilates is an excellent choice for people looking for a way of reducing the negative effects of emotional, mental and physical stress and tension without putting their bodies through a punishing exercise programme. It's also an excellent way of encouraging anyone to develop greater awareness and confidence in their bodies.

The Pilates approach is very demanding in terms of the exercises which must be done in an extremely controlled, precise way, but it does not encourage an unhealthily competitive approach to physical fitness. Apart from its stress-reducing potential, regular practice of Pilates exercises appears to promote a leaner, taller body shape, while encouraging stronger and more supple muscles and joints.

what to expect from a class

A Pilates class focuses on building core stability in the area of the torso (this extends roughly from the lower ribcage to the pelvic floor). The aim of working from this area is to create a 'girdle of strength' around your trunk to protect your spine and internal organs. As a result, you should find that this benefits your back in dramatically reducing back pain, improves your alignment and posture, and enables you to safely bend and twist. By consciously thinking about the beginning of each movement in this way before exercising, you are far less likely to strain or injure muscles. The latter can often happen when repetitions of exercises are done without paying attention and listening to your body.

The specific exercises, while not obviously very physical, like running and jumping, require a considerable focus and concentration in order to gain maximum benefit. This is because the movements involved are designed to work in a very intense way on isolated muscles groups. Although these movements may sometimes seem very small, do not be misled into thinking this is a soft option, since they may be held for a comparatively long period of time. As a result, a class should leave you feeling that you have worked quite hard and in a concentrated way.

The benefits attributed to regular Pilates exercises are impressive in their range. Positive effects include enhanced flexibility, improved mental and emotional balance, leaner, longer muscles, better muscle tone and strength, and improved postural alignment. Since the correct performance of these exercises demands a great deal of concentration and mental focus as well as coordination of breathing patterns, Pilates can also have a profound effect on reducing the negative effect of stress.

how does pilates work?

By concentrating on developing what is known as functional strength. Pilates exercises can encourage the body to become stronger without losing flexibility and optimum alignment. As a result, muscles should become leaner, longer and stronger without developing the muscle-bound look of a body builder. In contrast to other forms of exercise that focus on working the superficial muscles of the body, Pilates concentrates on muscles that are located at a deeper level. Pilates exercises also focus on lengthening muscles so that they are less likely to shorten and bulk up. This encourages flexibility as well as a more streamlined body shape.

This system of movement can be of particular benefit to anyone who has a high stress, sedentary lifestyle with a tendency to poor postural habits. Not only does Pilates hold out the possibility of better body posture, more flexible muscles and a leaner outline, it also focuses the mind on relaxing the body through controlled movements and coordinated breathing techniques.

creative therapies

spiritual healing

We can regard the general approach of healing as yet another way of encouraging the self-healing mechanism of the body to work more efficiently. There are many forms of healing, including the currently popular reiki, absent healing, faith healing, spiritual healing, therapeutic touch and aura healing. It is not necessary to have any religious or spiritual belief in order to consider some form of healing as a possible extra avenue of therapeutic support.

the first treatment

Much of what happens depends on the approach adopted by the individual practitioner. For instance, in therapeutic touch you may be asked to lie down or remain seated fully clothed while the therapist moves their hands over your body, locating the areas of energy flow that need attention. Other healers may choose to work with you sitting in a chair, with their hands slightly above your head.

Some therapists choose to create a tranquil, soothing atmosphere by using soft light, candles or discreet music, while others may be happy to visit you in your own home. Whatever the healer's approach, there appears to be general agreement that, for the most favourable results, the patient should be at ease with the way the healer works and feel a positive rapport with them.

This is not of course limited to healing since whatever therapy is being explored, there needs to be a favourable rapport between therapist and patient.

Research trials

Although there is no scientific explanation for what happens during or following a healing session, some interesting research has been done to date, suggesting that this field might merit further, more rigorous trials and assessment.

In 1993, an American healer, Dr Daniel Benor, undertook an ambitious review of 155 trials of healing, claiming that 60 per cent of the patients in the trials showed positive improvements in anxiety, high blood pressure and speedier healing of wounds. The British healer Matthew Manning has worked with scientists under laboratory conditions, with some results showing that he could influence biochemical changes in the contents of a laboratory flask. A controversial trial from the United States (conducted in San Francisco in the late 1980s) suggested that absent healing through prayer could promote positive results in patients recovering from surgery.

how does healing work?

Although, as yet, there is no way of demonstrating the mechanism by which healing works, practitioners often describe what they do as 'connecting' with healing energy. Loosely speaking, the object of healing is to help stimulate the body's self-healing potential. In order to stimulate this energy flow, healers hold or move their hands above or lightly on the body, sometimes making sweeping movements. They identify problem areas by sensations of heat or cold, and you too may feel changes in sensation during the course of a treatment. These include tingling, warmth or cold, or slight light-headedness. Some healers say that their hands feel warm during the course of a treatment, as they make contact with changes in the patient's energy field.

Conventional science still struggles with healing as a method of treatment, and some doctors suggest that any benefits are due to the placebo effect ('mind over matter'). However, even if this accounts for only a small degree of the improvement experienced by a patient, it may still be regarded as providing valuable psychological support, especially for patients struggling with chronic problems. Another explanation suggests that some of the benefits associated with healing techniques are due to changes in the brainwave patterns experienced by healer and recipient, which resemble those of people who meditate.

colour and crystal therapy

We are constantly surrounded by colour: each day we choose the colour of the clothes that we will wear and we often buy an object because we are attracted by its colour (this could be anything from a major purchase such as a car, to the paint we choose to decorate the walls of our homes). These choices can change according to the mood we happen to be in at any given time. Soothing, calming blue and greens are likely to be appealing at moments of tension and warm reds will be attractive at times when a boost of energy and passion is called for.

Although we may regard these choices as purely practical, exponents of colour therapy would argue otherwise. They suggest that the colours we find attractive give us important clues about our basic drives and hidden needs. One relatively recent form of colour therapy, which is increasing in popularity, is aura-soma. This combines the use of essential oils, plant extracts, crushed gems and crystals to create a range of vibrantly coloured liquids. The patient's choice of colours leads to diagnosis.

Healers use crystal therapy to balance the energy levels in the body. Gemstones, such as rose quartz, topaz and garnet, are thought to possess their own form of healing energy. A crystal therapist may suggest that you wear a crystal that has a particular therapeutic resonance for you around your neck or that you keep in your room to dispel negative energy around computers, for example.

the first treatment

During a colour therapy session your therapist will ask you to look at a collection of 102 bottles of coloured liquids illuminated by a light box. You will then be asked to select your first, second, third and fourth choice in order of attraction.

The therapist will then explain what these colour choices mean. The first relates to your purpose in life, the second to your gifts and talents, the third reflects where you are right now and the fourth relates to your future. The therapist may give you one of the bottles of coloured liquid to take away (especially if it relates to an area that presents you with some degree of challenge). They may encourage you to meditate while focusing your gaze on the colour of the liquid in the bottle, adding it to a soothing bath or applying it to certain areas of your body.

Apart from using your chosen bottles of coloured liquid at home, you may become more aware of the effect that certain colours have on you. If you are drawn to certain colours, it may be worth thinking about what these are saying about your needs at any given time.

Aura-soma therapy is thought to help minor psychological disturbances where the patient appreciates that colour choices can affect their mood. As a result, this therapy may be of help to anyone suffering from minor anxiety or stress symptoms. It can be combined with other more adjunctive therapies. Adjunctive essentially means those complementary therapies that can be used to support the action of each other – such as reflexology, flower essences, and/or healing.

how do colour and crystal therapies work?

There is no explanation of how colour and crystal therapies work and it is generally thought that these healing measures are best kept for the treatment of minor problems. Where more established or more severe health problems are concerned, it is important to bear in mind that more established therapies will probably be more appropriate.

The properties of colour

The following is a very basic guide to the properties of the principal colours:

• Red – linked to passion, confidence and energy.

• Yellow – uplifting and energy-boosting.

• Orange – can stimulate outgoing tendencies and boosts confidence.

• Green – primarily balancing, soothing and calming.

• Blue – associated with relaxation and tranquility.

• Indigo (or lighter shades such as violet or lavender) – can help induce a meditative state.

arts therapies

Many of us are instinctively aware that music, dance or visual arts can affect our mood. Arts therapies take this concept one step further by suggesting that we can tap into these creative activities and, as a result, improve our overall sense of health and well-being. Ideally, arts therapies encourage and allow us to connect with our creative side which may have lain dormant for many years and, in many cases, since childhood.

The main arts therapies are as follows:

Dance This can include specific types of dance such as flamenco or more free-flowing forms of self-expression, such as eurhythmy, a rhythmic system of body movement related to poetry and music created by Rudolf Steiner.

Painting This can involve the general therapeutic effect that comes from enjoying being part of a drawing or painting group, or more structured therapeutic work, where the artwork produced is considered to be a guide to emotional and psychological well-being.

Music This can involve active participation (such as learning how to sing or learning to play a musical instrument) or listening to music for its aesthetic as well as therapeutic effect.

first sessions

Arts therapy is a valuable tool in helping people of all ages safely to express feelings that may be leading to anxieties, conflicts and distress. Ideally this is best done with adequate psychological and/or psychiatric support. To start with, your therapist will assess your individual situation by asking about your overall medical history, including details of your emotional and psychological health.

You can expect to attend one session a week and for the session to last roughly 60–90 minutes. During this time, your arts therapist will encourage you to create a collage or painting, using your instincts as a guide. As they will make clear at the outset, the purpose of this exercise is not to create a 'perfect' art work but to allow you to express whatever emotions need to be expressed through colour, shape and form. It may take time and the gentle guidance of the therapist before you become sufficiently unselfconscious to be able to express yourself without self-criticism and self-censorship.

Dance classes can prove very therapeutic by allowing us to express frustration, anger, sadness, or any other emotions that we find difficult to connect with on a day-to-day basis. Giving ourselves up to the rhythm of a musical accompaniment can put us back in touch with our bodies in a way that is denied to us in our daily routine. As with other forms of movement, we may find that the dance form we choose to explore can energize or calm us, depending on our needs at the time.

Music can have a profound effect on mood and emotional well-being. Some fascinating studies recently have shown that listening to specific styles of music, such as the Baroque, can induce feelings of well-being and tranquillity, while more raucous, aggressive forms of music can induce or magnify feelings of negativity and/or mild depression. Clearly, our taste in music can vary from day to day according to our emotional needs. One day we are 'up' and may instinctively want to bask in sounds that make us feel chilled out and calm, while on other occasions we instinctively know that we need music that will lift our spirits and energize us. Singing or playing a musical instrument (in the same way as drawing or painting) can give us access to a powerful form of non-verbal communication. As a result, we may find that a close involvement and association with music can yield important emotional and psychological benefits in a most pleasurable way.

how do arts therapies work?

Most of these therapies appear to work by putting us in contact with emotions and feelings that are in need of a safe channel for expression. Music in particular appears to have the capacity to touch emotions that we may not otherwise be able to access easily. Dance, being very physical, brings with it all the benefits of aerobic exercise to mind and body, as well as allowing us to express emotions and creativity.

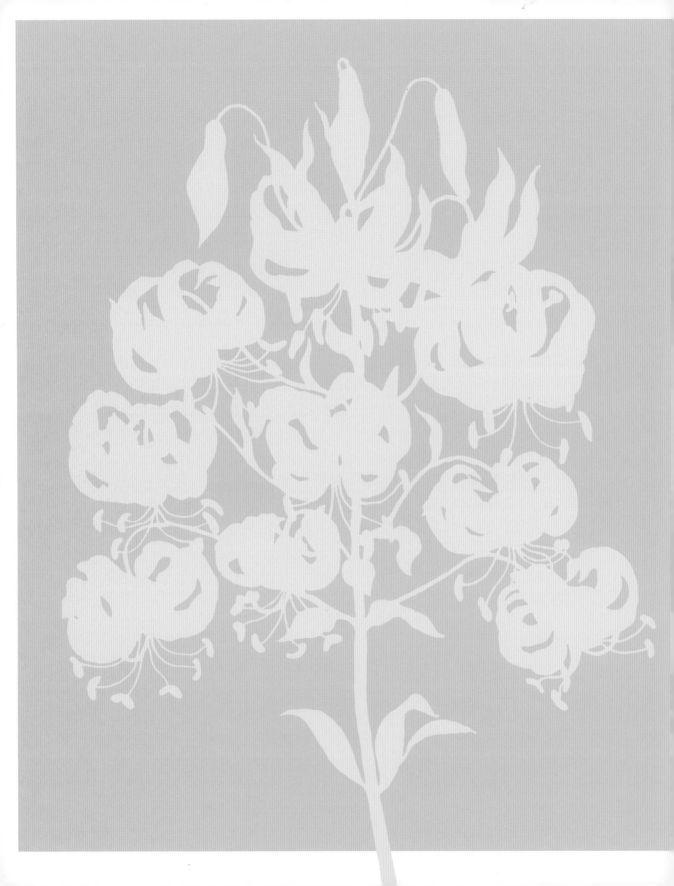

common ailments

introduction

Although the majority of the ailments selected for this book relate especially to women, others commonly occur in everyone. What they all have in common is their suitability for complementary treatment.

The ailments are grouped according to the area of the body which they affect. Each account includes a list of the common symptoms, an outline of the treatments usually offered by conventional medicine and more detailed descriptions of suitable complementary treatments, as well as certain practical measures that may improve the situation.

Self-treatment is not always advisable, in which case you should consult a practitioner of one of the complementary therapies listed. Most treatments can be used alongside conventional therapy and offer a valuable means of support.

contents

burn-out

Symptoms of burn-out, which may be immensely varied, are listed below. The problems of burn-out commonly set in after a period of high stress that has put mind and body under pressure. As a result, the body can become exhausted and less able to fight off infections effectively, while the mind can throw up symptoms of nervous exhaustion.

common symptoms

- **Extreme mental, emotional and physical fatigue**
- **Inability to cope with life and its demands**
- **Poor sleep pattern**
- **Digestive problems**
- **Aches and pains**
- **Recurrent headaches**
- **Low-grade infections**
- **Mood swings**
- **Difficulty in concentrating**
- **Inability to switch off mentally**
- **Raised pulse rate**
- **Withdrawal from relationships**
- **Chronic fatigue syndrome**

conventional treatments

It may be necessary to take time off work, ideally coupled with some form of stress-management counselling in order to prevent the situation recurring. If depression, anxiety and sleep disturbance are a problem, a doctor may prescribe a course of antidepressants.

complementary treatments

In the early stages, some of the following self-help measures may be sufficient to turn around the situation. However, if the situation is more established, or symptoms are severe, you should consult a registered practitioner.

aromatherapy

In the short term, essential oils derived from citrus fruits can help to boost flagging mental and physical energy levels, while lifting low mood. Inhale a few drops of grapefruit, orange or lemon essential oils from a tissue or evaporate them in a custom-made vaporizer.

homeopathy

Nux vomica This will almost certainly help classic mild to moderate burn-out dating from a stressful time at work and at home, or following a phase of 'burning the candle at both ends'. Symptoms include light, easily disturbed sleep with problems switching off, hangover-type headaches, indigestion and constipation, and a tendency to be on an emotional short fuse.

Lycopodium Use this for burn-out associated with anticipatory anxiety (such as worrying about meeting a deadline or giving a presentation at work). Characteristic symptoms include alternating bouts of diarrhoea and constipation, indigestion and heartburn.

Arsenicum album This may help mild to moderate symptoms of burn-out that emerge in pathological perfectionists and high achievers. Common symptoms include constant nausea from anxiety, poor sleep with a tendency to wake in the early hours feeling anxious and physical and mental restlessness.

nutritional approaches

• Avoid alcohol, coffee and fizzy drinks, chocolate, sticky pastries and junk foods.

• Instead, eat foods and drinks that help to stimulate high-level mental, emotional and physical health (and give yourself a boost into the bargain!). These include wholegrain foods; high-fibre foods, such as fresh fruit and vegetables (for slow, steady energy release); small amounts of high-quality protein, such as fish and organic, free-range poultry; and green tea, which is rich in anti-oxidants (which help our bodies fight infection) and low in caffeine.

• The nutrient Co-enzyme Q10 is known as 'the spark of life' because of its potential for balancing flagging energy levels and increasing antibody production, thus enabling the body to fight infections more effectively. Dietary sources include oily fish such as mackerel and sardines, as well as offal and peanuts. If you take supplements, aim for a dose of approximately 30 mg a day.

western herbalism

Take wild oats, ginseng or vervain in the form of infusions, capsules, or tinctures.
Warning Avoid vervain during pregnancy.

bach flower remedies

Elm can be a useful support where there is a tendency to take on an excessive workload that results in an overwhelming feeling of responsibility.

active therapies

Relaxation is one of the most effective routes to re-establishing healthy mental, emotional and physical energy levels. Consider meditation and guided visualization, progressive muscular relaxation or autogenic training, progressive muscular relaxation, yoga and tai chi.

insomnia

Strictly speaking, insomnia means a total inability to sleep but it usually includes a variety of disruptions to a healthy sleep pattern. Symptoms of poor sleep pattern vary and can include any combination of those listed below. Sleep disturbance can commonly follow looking after a young baby or nursing a sick relative, and can also be related to hormonal fluctuations. Many women also experience sleep problems pre-menstrually.

common symptoms

- Exhaustion on going to bed, but an inability to switch off
- Falling asleep quite quickly, but waking shortly afterwards (perhaps an hour or two) feeling ready to get up
- Waking around 5–6 am after a fitful, unrefreshing sleep
- Sleeping badly and waking feeling sleepy and unprepared to face the day ahead
- Waking early but falling into a deep sleep when it is time to get up

conventional treatments

Nowadays, doctors may suggest a short course of sleeping tablets or tranquillizers to break a temporary cycle of sleeplessness or anxiety. If this fails to solve the problem, the next step may be a course of antidepressants that have a sedative-type effect.

complementary treatments

Any of the self-help measure below may help to relive insomnia or poor sleep. The beauty of complementary treatments is that they seldom bring side effects and never bring concerns about dependency in their wake. As a result, they can be used safely to break a recent cycle of poor quality or disturbed sleep in a gentle, but effective way.

aromatherapy

Add a few drops of lavender, chamomile, frankincense, ylang ylang or mandarin essential oils to your bath for a soothing and relaxing soak.

Warning Avoid chamomile and frankincense during pregnancy.

homeopathy

Nux vomica This is one of the first remedies to consider when sleep has been disrupted by stress, especially if you have increased your consumption of caffeine, alcohol and/or cigarettes in an effort to keep up with the pace.

Arsenicum album Use this to ease symptoms of anxiety that emerge with particular force in the small hours of the morning, causing such physical and emotional restlessness that it feels impossible to get to sleep. When this remedy is needed, warm, soothing drinks help.

Lachesis This may reduce fear of going to bed because of the prospect of lying awake for hours. It is also a key remedy for creative people who find themselves buzzing with ideas in the early hours of the morning.

nutritional approaches

Avoid drinks containing caffeine last thing at night. Caffeine is a stimulant and makes it more difficult to switch off and drift into a restful slumber. Make it a rule not to drink strong coffee, cocoa, tea, or alcohol after 4 pm.

naturopathy

• This simple hydrotherapy technique may help you drift off to sleep more soundly. Take a pair of cotton socks, immerse them in cool water and wring them out thoroughly. Put the damp socks on your feet and put thicker, dry woollen socks over the top of them. Get into a warm bed before you get chilled, which would stop you from getting comfortably relaxed and rested.

Warning Anyone suffering from circulatory problems should not have hydrotherapy.

• Finish work at least a couple of hours before going to bed in order to make it easier to switch off.

• Avoid eating heavy meals late at night, which makes it much harder to sleep properly.

western herbalism

A recent study conducted at Northumbria University in the United Kingdom showed impressive responses to lemon balm. Valerian, passiflora and wild oats can also help us drift into a sound, restorative sleep. These come in the form of tinctures, tablets or teas.

bach flower remedies

White chestnut is especially helpful in situations of sleeplessness where thoughts keep buzzing relentlessly through the mind, preventing it from switching off.

addictions

In our 'quick-fix' society, it is not surprising to find a wide range of addictions. These can vary from a low-grade dependence to apparently innocuous substances, such as sugar and caffeine, to more serious addictions such as those to alcohol, cigarettes, and prescription and recreational drugs. In additon, there are behavioural addictions such as gambling.

common symptoms

- **Mood swings**
- **Irritability**
- **Lack of concentration**
- **Fatigue**
- **Poor sleep pattern**
- **Anxiety**
- **Depression**
- **Digestive problems, such as lack of appetite, nausea and/or food cravings**

conventional treatments

Major problems of alcohol and drug addiction require professional treatment in the form of psychological support, drug therapy and controlled withdrawal programmes. These help the patient to come to terms with and move on from their addiction. Giving up smoking, which has more long-term consequences, may be helped by nicotine patches.

complementary treatments

For minor problems of addiction (such as caffeine or sugar dependency) the following complementary advice can be helpful in making the break and getting back on a healthy track again.

aromatherapy

Any of the following essential oils can be used in massage blends (diluted in a carrier oil), added to a warm bath, or vaporized in an oil burner.

• Fennel and juniper (for detoxifying)

• Bergamot, clary sage, chamomile and ylang ylang (to balance or lift mood)

homeopathy

Nux vomica This can give exceptional support when giving up caffeine, cigarettes or alcohol. This is especially indicated if symptoms include classic 'hangover' headaches, queasiness, constipation and problems in getting into a refreshing sleep at night. Irritability and being on an emotional 'short fuse' are also likely to be striking features.

Argenticum nitricum (Arg. nit.)
Nervous exhaustion resulting from high stress levels and on-going anxiety states, coupled with a craving for sugar (which, in the long term, aggravates digestive problems) respond better to this remedy.

nutritional approaches

Supplements of vitamins A, C, D and B complex, and manganese and potassium can give essential support to the body during withdrawal.

naturopathy

• To avoid unpleasant symptoms of caffeine withdrawal (such as jitteriness, headaches and a general washed-out feeling), it is best not to give up suddenly. Instead, gradually reduce the number of daily cups of caffeinated drinks, steadily introducing caffeine-free alternatives such as grain-based coffee substitutes and herbal or fruit teas.

• Switching to the odd cup of weak green tea can also be helpful, since it is rich in health-promoting anti-oxidants that help support the body's defences.

• Drink at least four large glasses of filtered tap water or still mineral water each day. This will help the body flush out toxic waste, while helping to prevent any symptoms of low-grade dehydration, such as fatigue, constipation and headaches.

western herbalism

• Milk thistle has a particularly beneficial, regenerative effect on the liver and can be taken either as an infusion or as 5 ml of diluted tincture three times a day.
Warning Avoid during pregnancy or in large doses.

• Dandelion can also help in detoxifying the body, especially if there is a tendency to fluid retention.
Warning Avoid dandelion if you have gall bladder problems.

• Wild oats can be especially helpful if addiction to coffee, cigarettes or prescription drugs such as painkillers containing codeine has developed in response to excess emotional stress and tension. Take 8 drops of tincture diluted in a small glass of water twice a day.

bach flower remedies

When the pressure is on and you miss that shot of caffeine and/or cigarette, try Rescue Remedy. In a tight spot, place a few drops under the tongue or, when more time is available, dissolve the recommended number of drops suggested on the label of the bottle in a small glass of water. Take a sip as and when required.

hypnotherapy

This can be a helpful avenue of support when trying to kick the habit of smoking cigarettes.

anxiety

Long-term anxiety can give rise to very unpleasant emotional and physical symptoms such as those listed below. We can be more prone to anxiety at times of high stress or hormonal upheaval, for example, pre-menstrually or leading up to or during menopause. Anxiety can also accompany an episode of depression, with symptoms alternating between feeling 'blue' and agitated and jittery.

common symptoms

- Palpitations (rapid or fluttering heartbeat)
- Nausea
- Diarrhoea
- Loss of appetite (or sometimes comfort eating)
- Perspiration
- Loss of sleep
- Lack of concentration
- Mood swings
- Headaches
- Trembling

conventional treatments

For short-term anxiety with an obvious cause, these usually involve the prescription of antidepressants that also have a sedative effect. More established or severe episodes of anxiety may respond well to counselling or psychological approaches, such as cognitive behavioural therapy (CBT). Beta blockers may be another possible avenue of support through conventional treatments.

complementary treatments

Any of the following measures would be excellent for any short-term episode of anxiety. However, for severe and/or well-established anxiety, you should consult an experienced practitioner.

practicalities

Aerobic exercise can be immensely helpful in creating a natural tranquillizing effect (with none of the drawbacks of chemical sedatives). According to the Exercise Laboratory of California, a brisk walk may reduce anxiety as effectively as a 400 mg dose of a tranquilizer. Good examples of aerobic exercise are cycling, running, 'power walking' and dancing.

aromatherapy

Inhale a drop or two of lavender, geranium, clary sage or neroli essential oil from a tissue to reduce anxiety when under pressure.

homeopathy

Arsenicum album Use this for anxiety that keeps you awake at night. It is especially indicated for minor or short-term anxiety symptoms in anyone who is a perfectionist, which is often accompanied by nausea and/or diarrhoea.

Lycopodium This may ease the anxiety, often accompanied by digestive disturbances, that sets in before speaking in public or being the focus of attention.

Aconite Use this to ease the anxiety that triggers panic attacks, in which feelings of sheer terror descend out of the blue, accompanied by a genuine fear that it will be impossible to survive the attack.

nutritional approaches

Limit your caffeine intake, since this can aggravate symptoms of anxiety such as palpitations, mood swings and insomnia. Avoid drinking more than two cups of caffeinated drinks a day (not forgetting that fizzy colas can have a hefty dose of caffeine added to them).

naturopathy

• Use calming breathing techniques to banish feelings of panic and anxiety, checking that you are breathing correctly (see page 10).

western herbalism

Opt for soothing, calming herbal teas such as chamomile. If the taste of chamomile does not appeal, choose one of the naturally tranquillizing blends of herbal teas available. The ingredients to look for are valerian, passiflora and lemon balm.

bach flower remedies

• General anxiety, with fears of the unknown and a general sense of foreboding may be eased by aspen.

• A specific anxiety about losing control may be helped by cherry plum.

yoga

Regular practice of yoga is also beneficial. Well known for its mood-balancing, calming effect and for promoting a leaner, stronger, more flexible body, yoga also focuses on the need to breathe deeply and rhythmically. In this way, you gain the most from the postures while also harmonizing the mind and body.

panic attacks

These extremely unsettling and alarming episodes can be an unpleasant feature of anxiety. They may occur as a one-off or episodically. The first panic attack may be so terrifying that we feel certain that we are about to die. However, if this should ever happen, remember that no one has been known to die of a panic attack. Once you know how to take action, this will help you feel more in control and better able to cope.

common symptoms

- **Rapid heartbeat**
- **Sweating**
- **Nausea and/or diarrhoea**
- **Breathlessness**
- **Feeling faint, light-headed, dizzy or disoriented**

conventional treatments

Nowadays, doctors seldom prescribe tranquillizers as a first resort because of the problems with dependency. Instead, they may prescribe drugs such as beta blockers or antidepressants that have a sedative effect for use in the short term, or offer counselling or cognitive therapy for more long-term help.

complementary treatments

Any of the following therapies can be used as effective, practical avenues of support in order to help us get through a panic attack in the shortest time possible, with the least amount of distress. For longer-term help in dealing with symptoms of severe and/or long-established anxiety, consult an experienced practitioner.

naturopathy

Calming breathing techniques can be pivotal in getting through a panic attack as swiftly as possible. At the first sign of uneasiness, try to relax your jaw and facial muscles, allowing your shoulders to drop a few inches away from your ears. Take steady, full breaths, making sure that the in-breath is equal to the out-breath. Counting slowly as your breathe in and out may help you focus your mind.

western herbalism

Sipping a cup of lemon balm tea can be immensely soothing to jangled, frayed nerves because of its gentle tranquillizing effect on the nervous system.

bach flower remedies

Rescue Remedy is available in an easy-to-use spray form that can be kept in a handbag and used at the first sign of a panic attack. Follow the dosage instructions on the container.

hyperventilation

Whenever we feel tense and anxious, our natural inclination is to breathe quickly and shallowly from the top of the chest rather than the diaphragm. This increase the uptake of oxygen which can lead to the symptoms listed below. The trick is to know how to breathe consciously in a relaxed way so that the pattern of breathing can be changed to help you calm down.

common symptoms

- **Dizziness**
- **Palpitations**
- **Perspiration**
- **Increased feelings of panic and agitation**

conventional treatments

Unless the problem is associated with asthma, treatment usually involves drugs such as beta blockers, which calm feelings of panic as well as treating high blood pressure. Relaxation techniques or counselling may also be advisable.

complementary treatments

A trained practitioner is likely to focus on exploring the underlying issues that are causing tension and anxiety. However, the following suggestions may be helpful in the short-term for the occasional bout of hyperventilation.

aromatherapy

Vaporize a few drop of geranium oil or inhale it from a tissue. This helps to calm the nervous system, so will help to calm panic-related rapid breathing.

homeopathy

Aconite This can quickly ease hyper-ventilation linked to feelings of anxiety. One or two tablets taken at the first sign of trouble should work within minutes.

naturopathy

We tend to take breathing for granted, only thinking about it when something seems to be amiss. If you tend to breathe quickly when stressed, take slow, deep breaths, using the whole of your lung capacity from the top to the bottom. In this way, you will balance the levels of oxygen and carbon dioxide in the blood, which will help you to calm down.

bach flower remedies

Always have a bottle of Rescue Remedy to hand if occasional hyperventilation is a problem when you are under pressure. Place a few drops under the tongue or dilute the recommended number of drops in a glass of water.

depression

The symptoms of mild to moderate depression are wide-ranging, but relatively easy to spot. It is commonly a reaction to stress, bereavement or personal problems such as divorce or money worries or failed relationships. More serious types of depression may be biochemical in origin and are beyond the scope of this book. Symptoms are listed below.

common symptoms

- **Low mood with uncharacteristic feelings of apathy and indifference**
- **Negativity and pessimism about life**
- **Lack of appetite or binge-eating fuelled by a need for comfort**
- **Poor sleep pattern with a tendency to wake in the early hours feeling jittery and depressed**
- **Lack of confidence**
- **Reduced libido**
- **Poor concentration and memory**
- **Abrupt mood changes**

Warning: Established or severe problems with depression need professional medical attention

conventional treatments

Where an episode of depression is related to a traumatic event (such as bereavement, relationship break-up or stress at work), a doctor may prescribe antidepressants and also recommend psychological support in the form of counselling or cognitive behavioural therapy. If it's not reactive depression it would fall into a category of clinical (called endogenous) depression which is likely to need more skilled treatment from a specialist such as a psychiatrist. Some doctors may be skilled enough to deal with the situation, but many take a more generalist stance.

complementary treatments

A mild bout of depression triggered by a specific event (or a series of stressful episodes) may respond well to some of the self-help measures outlined below.

practicalities

Regular, rhythmic exercise that gets the heart, lungs and large muscles of the legs moving can help lift a mild low mood. For optimum mood-balancing effect, aim for a regular work-out. Three or four 30-minute sessions each week are better than one 2-hour session every week or so.

aromatherapy

Dilute chamomile, clary sage, lavender, marjoram, ylang ylang, bergamot, geranium or jasmine essential oils in a carrier oil in order to make a mood-balancing massage blend. Alternatively, vaporize a few drops in an oil-burner or add a few drops to warm bathwater for a soothing soak.

homeopathy

Natrum muriaticum (Natrum mur.)
This may ease a withdrawn depression resulting from emotional trauma where feelings of sadness and distress have been suppressed. Common symptoms include a strong dislike of sympathy and affection, with an accompanying aversion to breaking down into tears,which is seen as humiliating rather than a healthy release of emotion.

Staphysagria This may have a positive effect on depression triggered by feelings of anger that have turned inward and festered rather than being expressed freely. It can be especially helpful in easing blues after invasive surgery or a high-tech birth, where there may be a lingering feeling of violation.

Sepia Use this to help episodes of depression linked to hormonal fluctuations, such as the onset of periods, pre-menstrual syndrome, after pregnancy and leading up to or during menopause. Characteristic features include complete mental, emotional and physical exhaustion, loss of sex drive, irritability and snappishness, with a feeling of being overwhelmed by responsibilities.

nutritional approaches

Avoid alcohol whenever possible because of its mood-enhancing effect. This may be fine on a fun night out, when we are feeling generally positive, but it can have the reverse effect when we are feeling low, making us feel even more negative after a few drinks.

western herbalism

Recent studies published in the *British Medical Journal* have shown St John s Wort (*Hypericum*) to be potentially effective in the treatment of mild to moderate depression.
Warning St John s Wort may reduce the effectiveness of some conventional drugs. Always consult your pharmacist or doctor before beginning self-treatment with St John s Wort.

bach flower remedies

Willow may ease the depressive feelings characterized by feelings of resentment and bitterness, together with an overwhelming sense of the unfairness of life.

'baby blues'

Getting physically and emotionally back on track after the birth of a baby can feel like riding a roller-coaster. One minute everything seems marvellous, while the next, you can feel totally down in the dumps. This is not surprising because hormone levels at this time are in turmoil and feelings about loss of freedom, inadequacy and new responsibilities can be overwhelming.

common symptoms

- Feeling overwhelmed, tearful and unable to cope with everyday demands
- Uncharacteristic feelings of indifference or complete lack of motivation
- Negativity or despair on waking
- Physical, mental and/or emotional exhaustion that is not lifted at all by periods of rest or relaxation

conventional treatments

Once the problem has been identified, support will probably take the form of short-term use of antidepressants and counselling or cognitive behavioural therapy (CBT). Post-natal depression is a more intense form of baby blues that definitely needs professional medical help and is outside the remit of responsible self-prescribing alone.

Warning If at any time you feel like harming yourself or your baby consult your doctor as soon as possible.

complementary treatments

If the baby blues descend soon after birth and it seems impossible to regain any sense of emotional balance, it is worth trying one of the following complementary treatments. However, if symptoms are slow to respond, or show signs of getting worse, do not be afraid to call on professional support. This can take the form of a consultation with a complementary therapist, counselling sessions or short-term support from conventional medication.

aromatherapy

Make a mood-balancing aromatic massage blend by adding 4 drops each of Roman chamomile, rose and ginger to 4 teaspoonsful of carrier oil. Use this to massage the body twice a day.
Warning Avoid if breastfeeding.

homeopathy

Natrum muriaticum (Natrum mur.)
This may lift a very withdrawn and low mood where there is a tendency to avoid displays of sympathy or emotion because they feel embarrassing.

Sepia This may help a mother who is feeling low and exhausted soon after birth and has problems emotionally bonding with her baby. Common feelings include apathy, indifference, lowered libido, a general sense of being unable to cope, and an overall fear of losing control.

Staphisagria This can be especially helpful in balancing roller-coaster moods, especially after a particularly hi-tech or Caesarian birth. These can leave the mother feeling violated by intrusive medical procedures or disappointed and angry if she had hoped for a natural birth.

nutritional approaches

• Avoid dietary items that aggravate mood swings and depression. These include alcohol, strong tea and coffee, sweets and fizzy drinks that are laced with caffeine and/or sugar. Opt instead for wholegrains, lots of fresh fruit and vegetables, and small portions of high-quality protein such as fish or poultry.

• Certain essential nutrients are associated with depressive feelings so you might consider taking supplements of vitamin B complex, vitamin C, magnesium and zinc.

naturopathy

Lack of exposure to sunlight diversely affects serotonin levels (a neurotransmitter responsible for maintaining healthy emotional balance). Since lack of sunshine also adversely affects the secretion of the female sex hormone oestrogen (which can also have a profound effect on mood), a daily stroll in the open air clearly has real benefits.

western herbalism

• An infusion of lemon balm can help lift a low mood or calm feelings of mild depression coupled with anxiety.

Steep 10 g lemon balm in a cup of hot water, strain and drink up to three times a day.

• For mild to moderate depression, consider St Johns Wort (*Hypericum*). For more details see Depression (pages 82–83). If breastfeeding, seek the advice of a trained medical herbalist rather than self-medicating.

bach flower remedies

• Olive can raise the spirits when there is a general sense of mental, emotional and physical burn-out and exhaustion.

• Wild rose can be helpful where feelings of indifference make motivation and focus a real problem.

bereavement

The support of friends and family can be invaluable in coming to terms with grief. It helps to be aware of the symptoms of grief and the order in which they happen, however, which can vary from one person to another. Remember that if you feel you are coping and slowly moving on, you don't automatically need to seek complementary help. But should you feel 'overwhelmed' or 'stuck', it's time to seek support.

feelings and common symptoms

- **An initial sense of unreality or unacceptance, especially if the death has been totally unexpected and shocking**
- **Guilt coupled with a sense of not having done enough to change the situation**
- **Anger, which is often focused on the person who has died**
- **Lack of apppetite**
- **Nausea**
- **Disturbed sleep patterns and sleep quality**

conventional treatments

In the short-term, a doctor may suggest a course of sedatives to give additional support during the period immediately after a death. For more long-term support, grief-counselling may be helpful because it gives the bereaved a chance to talk through painful emotions.

complementary treatments

Alternative and complementary approaches have a huge amount to offer in helping someone gently come to terms with the different phases of grieving. The advantage of complementary medicines and treatments is that they are not habit-forming and so there is no risk of addiction or dependence.

aromatherapy

Add a few drops of jasmine, bergamot, clary sage, neroli and rose essential oils to the bathwater for an emotionally restorative soak, or inhale the blend by applying a drop or two to a tissue. This combination may help relieve the emotional trauma that is part and parcel of the grieving process.

homeopathy

Ignatia This can have very positive effects on unresolved grief that does not seem to be shifting, however much time and support is at hand. This shows itself by abrupt changes in mood – from happy to sad within seconds – and much sighing, hiccuping or nervous twitching of the muscles as a result of holding in a lot of emotional tension.

Aconite Primarily a remedy for physical and emotional shock, this can be useful in the early stages of bereavement. It can be used for panic attacks that have lingered since hearing the news of a death and for severe, fast-developing symptoms of anxiety, restlessness and agitation.

Natrum muriaticum (Natrum mur.) Use this in the later stage of grieving, where emotions have been suppressed rather than allowed to surface. It is especially helpful for people who take a 'stiff upper lip' approach and who generally feel much worse for sympathy or a hug in case they burst into tears and humiliate themselves in front of everyone.

Staphysagria This is aimed at grieving that has got stuck at the anger stage, where the bereaved has hostility towards the person who has died and abandoned them, mixed with personal guilt and self-reproach at not having done enough.

nutritional approaches

Eat plenty of foods that contain B vitamins, because these are reputed to support the nervous system in times of extreme stress. Good sources include nuts, whole grains, green leafy vegetables, fish, yeast extract, soya flour, bananas and brown rice.

western herbalism

• To ease the feelings of shock accompanying bereavement, sip an infusion made from chamomile, lemon balm and skullcap whenever you feel on edge. This can also be a useful support when discontinuing tranquillizers after short-term use.

• A soothing infusion of borage may ease the feelings of tension, anxiety and palpitations that follow the shock of bereavement. Take it no more than three times daily and for no longer than 3 weeks at a time.

Warning This may have a negative effect on the liver if taken for too long or in too large a quantity.

bach flower remedies

Rescue Remedy can provide gentle, effective emotional support at difficult times and can be a support in both the early and later stages of grieving.

eating disorders

Women have an increasing reputation for having an uneasy love/hate relationship with food which is highlighted when problems with eating disorders develop. These disorders can take the form of anorexia (a fear of and aversion to eating), bulimia (compulsive over-eating and often self-induced vomiting) or binge-eating. Symptoms vary and can include any of those listed below.

commom symptoms

- **Strict reduction of the amount of food eaten each day**
- **Excessive monitoring of weight, to the extent of weighing several times a day**
- **Long-term dental problems caused by teeth being repeatedly bathed in stomach acid during vomiting**
- **An obsessive relationship with food, especially those regarded as 'forbidden' or dangerous due to their concentrated calorific content**
- **Using laxatives to reduce body weight**
- **Vomiting after binge eating**
- **Going on extreme diets such as those involving only one type of food**
- **Hormonal imbalances that cause a growth of extra body hair, diminished or arrested sex drive, and/or reduction in breast and hip contours**
- **Stopping of regular periods**

conventional treatments

A great deal depends on the stage and severity of the eating disorder when it is diagnosed. In very severe cases of anorexia, where the situation is life-threatening, admission to hospital for rehydration and artificial feeding may be necessary. Cases of bulimia may be helped by psychiatric support and specialized counselling.

Less severe cases may be referred for counselling and/or psychiatric help in order to try to deal with the underlying psychological issues that may be leading to the eating disorder. Where psychiatric help is given, conventional drugs may also be suggested.

complementary treatments

These may be helpful in milder cases where eating disorders are of a very low grade (for instance, where there is a history of 'yo-yo' dieting). In such a situation, the practitioner will probably want to explore some of the issues that may be triggering the problem. Since eating disorders can be potentially serious, it is best to seek help from a trained therapist rather than attempting self-treatment. The following suggestions may be used in addition to alternative, complementary and conventional medical help.

homeopathy

Arsenicum album This remedy may relieve any uneasy feelings about food, such as a fear of being sick as a result of the food being 'off'. It is suitable for high achievers and perfectionists, or people whose anxieties centre on food issues, with symptoms being worst at night.

Natrum muriaticum (Natrum mur.) This can help eating disorders stemming from unexpressed grief or emotional trauma, such as complete loss of appetite, or cravings for fatty, salty or starchy foods. Skin tone is likely to suffer, with a tendency to dry, tight skin on the face and cracking around the lips, possibly with outbreaks of cold sores.

Lycopodium Use this remedy for eating disorders arising from an excessive desire for control. This often occurs in hard-pressed people with a history of stress-related digestive problems, such as heartburn, acid reflux, bloating and/or alternating diarrhoea and constipation.

nutritional approaches

• Consult a nutritional specialist to see whether zinc deficiency is a problem. There appears to be a strong link between low zinc levels in the body and an increased tendency to eating disorders. Good sources of zinc include green vegetables, eggs, milk, whole grains, nuts, seeds, and meat.

• Add small, nutritious additional helpings of food at mealtimes and eat small, healthy snacks, such as raw, scrubbed vegetables, pieces of fresh fruit, or rice cakes made from organic brown rice to which savoury toppings can be added.

headaches and migraines

While headaches and migraine have certain symptoms in common, it is important to appreciate the differences between them. This is not just a question of degree of pain and the symptoms may include any of those listed below. Most headaches are not serious but medical advice is needed if they are accompanied by any unusual symptoms.

commmom symptoms

Migraine

- **Visual disturbance in one or both eyes**
- **Nausea and/or vomiting**
- **Severe, sickening pain on one side of the head or all over the head**
- **Disorientation, often with a tingling in the face or down one side of the body**
- **A lingering feeling of being unwell for a day or so after the pain has lifted**

Headaches

- **Tension headaches with tightness in the neck, jaw, scalp and shoulders**
- **'Cluster' headaches involving sporadic one-sided pain that lasts for a few hours or days**
- **Stabbing headaches**

Warning: If a headache is related to a severe blow to the head, or if is accompanied by clumsiness or a rash, seek urgent medical attention.

conventional treatments

Simple tension headaches can be treated with painkillers, but migraines may require special pain-relieving drugs that must be taken as soon as possible in order to gain relief. Occasionally, a doctor may prescribe beta blockers or a low dose of a tricyclic antidepressant.

complementary treatments

These tend to be equally well placed to deal with headaches or migraines. Any of the following self-help measures may ease an acute headache or migraine.

aromatherapy

Ease tension headaches and migraines by putting 1 drop of peppermint essential oil onto a cottonwool bud and applying it gently all along the hairline. If inhaling is easier, add 2 drops to a handkerchief or tissue and hold close to, but not touching, the nose.

homeopathy

Bryonia This can ease throbbing headaches which are made worse by the slightest movement and proportionally eased by keeping still.

Nux vomica This is suitable for classic 'morning after'-type headaches, easing any feeling of queasiness, noticeable constipation, sensitivity to noise and an emotional 'short fuse'.

Lachesis Use this to soothe migraines or headaches that come on after sleep (especially as the onset of a period gets closer). In these, pains settle above the left eye or move from left to right, with feelings of dizziness and disorientation.

massage

Regular neck and shoulder massage can help loosen up tight muscles in the areas that may be triggering tension headaches. Scalp massage can also be immensely relaxing, while making us aware of just how much tension we may be holding in this area.

osteopathy and chiropractic

Headaches often result from neck or shoulder tension, so osteopathy or chiropractic can be helpful in loosening up these areas and correcting any misalignment that may be contributing to the problem.

nutritional approaches

Avoid foods such as red wine, cheese, coffee and chocolate, which have a reputation for triggering migraines, especially when you feel low or under stress. Headaches can be caused by hunger or dehydration. A detox juice can help with headaches caused by a hangover.

western herbalism

• Drink a cup of meadowsweet tea three times a day. Infuse 1 teaspoonful of the herb in a cup of boiling water and strain it before drinking. The aspirin-type compounds found in the flowers and leaves help soothe a headache.

• According to research conducted in the 1980s, feverfew has a positive track record for treating migraines. Use it preventively by eating 2–3 fresh leaves between two slices of bread or take it in capsule form (following the recommended dose on the instructions).

lack of concentration

Loss of the ability to focus and concentrate can happen for a number of reasons. Common triggers are listed below. One of the most common triggers for a recently occurring problem with concentration and mental focus is unmanaged, high negative stress levels. If this is the case, taking stress management techniques on board wil pay huge dividends.

commom triggers

- **Lack of sound, refreshing sleep**
- **Unstable blood sugar levels**
- **Anxiety**
- **Depression**
- **Excessive stress levels that are not eased by stress management techniques**
- **Distracting background worries such as financial problems**
- **Pre-menstrual syndrome**
- **Menopause**
- **Attention Deficit Disorder (ADD)**

conventional treatments

Lack of concentration may be the result of an underlying problem, such as anxiety (see pages 78–79) or depression (see pages 82–83). On the other hand, if it seems to be related more to lack of stress management during a phase of very high negative tension, it may be more appropriate to look at psychological ways of managing the problem.

complementary treatments

If short-term poor concentration is linked to struggling with high stress levels, a complementary approach is likely to focus on ways of reducing the stress load on the mind and body through dietary, relaxation and exercise advice, as well as suggesting short-term techniques for focusing the mind.

aromatherapy

Inhale a drop or two of grapefruit, rosemary, peppermint or lemon essential oils from a tissue or vaporize them in an oil-burner.

homeopathy

Lycopodium This can ease lack of concentration arising from the anticipation of a challenging event, such as giving a public presentation. Once the event is underway, concentration levels return to their usual, excellent levels.

Nux vomica This may be effective when high stress levels are interfering with the ability to focus and concentrate. Lack of concentration goes hand in hand with a mental and emotional 'short fuse', along with a need for peace and quiet. This remedy also acts on any craving for coffee or other caffeinated drinks that can interfere with, rather than enhance, concentration levels.

nutritional approaches

• Recent French research suggests that the supplement Ginko biloba plays an important role in mental functioning by improving blood flow to the brain. The recommended dose is 30–50 mg three times daily but it is advisable to wait 3 months before evaluating its effects. In other words, do not be disappointed if there is no immediate improvement.

• Zinc is also thought to play an important role in keeping the mind sharp and focused, while especially enhancing memory. Approximately 50 per cent of the population in the United Kingdom are thought to be zinc-deficient to some degree. The recommended daily intake is 15 mg but, according to some government surveys, the average intake is more like 7.6 mg a day. Excellent dietary sources of zinc include seeds, peas, beans, lentils, nuts, meat and fish, including oysters.

naturopathy

Good quality sleep on a regular basis ensures that we will be full of mental, emotional and physical energy during the day, as well as being able to focus mentally. Studies have repeatedly shown that extended periods of sleep deprivation leads to increased mood swings, irritability, anxiety and poor concentration.

bach flower remedies

Flower essences with a positive reputation for encouraging mental focus under pressure include larch, elm, white chestnut, hornbeam, gentian and clematis. These can be taken either separately or together in a convenient custom-made blend.

meditation

Learning how to meditate can be a very positive step towards sharpening up levels of concentration. Meditation gives the mind a much-needed rest, so a regular session should enable us to deal with life's challenges much more effectively.

eye strain

Regular problems with eye strain can be an early warning sign that some aspects of your lifestyle need to be improved. Symptoms include 'tired' eyes, dryness and irritability. Common triggers of eye strain are listed below. If recurrent headaches are becoming a noticeable feature of life, this can also suggest that your eyes would benefit from being examined.

common triggers

- **Reading and/or working in conditions of poor light**
- **Lack of sound, refreshing sleep**
- **Neglecting regular eye examinations**
- **Working for long periods at a computer screen with no regular breaks**
- **Eye make-up**
- **Light intolerance, especially when working under artificial lighting**

conventional treatments

Regular eye examinations are very important once you reach the age of 40 years, after which the eyes tend to change and reading glasses are often necessary. However, anyone suffering from eye strain on a regular basis, especially if it is triggering headaches, should visit an optician. They may advise reading glasses or, if you already wear glasses, a change of prescription. If the eyes are chronically dry, eye drops that act as artificial tears may be necessary.

complementary treatments

Any of the following self-help measures may be used in addition to regular checks by your optician.

practicalities

If your eyes seem strained and tired, make sure that you are not aggravating the problem by using eye make-up to which you may be sensitive. If you suspect that this may be the case, switch to allergy-free products and be sure to remove all traces of eye make-up before going to bed.

aromatherapy

If eye strain is related to difficulty in switching off when your head hits the pillow, try a relaxing, warm bath an hour or so before bed. Add 5 drops of lavender essential oil to a soothing bath to encourage both mind and body to relax.

Warning Never use aromatherapy oils near the eyes because of the extremely delicate and sensitive skin in this area.

homeopathy

Ruta This can ease the feeling of tiredness and strain around the eyes that occurs after reading for too long.

nutritional approaches

If lack of sleep is making your eyes feel strained and tired, reduce your caffeine intake to no more than two cups a day and avoid it altogether during the second half of the day. Remember that there is caffeine in colas and high-energy fizzy drinks as well as tea and coffee.

naturopathy

• If you read a lot at work, get into the habit of refocusing your eyes every 20 minutes or so. To do this, look away from whatever you are concentrating on and focus on a point in the distance for roughly half a minute.

• Learn some exercises to strengthen your eye muscles. The best-known system is the Bates method and your optician can advise you about this.

• Make a point of blinking regularly when reading in order to lubricate the eyes.

western herbalism

If your develop short-term eye strain after working extra-long hours or driving under demanding conditions, give your eyes a treat by placing a wrung-out, cool chamomile teabag over each eye. Lie down for 10 minutes, with your feet up, listening to some relaxing music.

conjunctivitis

This irritating eye condition develops when the conjunctiva that covers the surface of the eyes and lines the eyelids becomes inflamed. Common triggers include bacterial or viral infection or an allergic reaction. Bacterial infections tend to affect both eyes, while a viral infection is more likely to affect one eye. Common symptoms are listed below.

common symptoms

- **Discomfort and 'grittiness' of the eyes**
- **A red, bloodshot look to the whites of the eyes that is worse away from the iris**
- **A pus-like discharge forming a yellowish crust that sticks the eyelids together overnight**
- **Puffiness around the eye**
- **Recurrent irritation, inflammation and/or itching of the eye**
- **Redness of the whites of the eye**
- **Sensitivity, especially during the hay fever season. This is specifically related to an allergic reaction.**

Warning: If symptoms continue to develop, or if you have severe pain in only one eye, see your doctor immediately.

conventional treatments

Doctors usually treat bacterial conjunctivitis with antibiotic cream or antibiotic drops, which you apply to the eye and eyelids, and they may also advise you how to avoid spreading the infection, by not sharing face cloths or hand towels. They may suggest moisturizing eye drops to soothe viral or allergic conjunctivitis.

complementary treatments

These can be used at the first sign of conjunctivitis to soothe discomfort and inflammation. If you suffer from conjunctivitis on a fairly regular basis, and if it seems to be linked to hay fever or allergic rhinitis, treatment by a complementary or alternative practitioner may be most helpful.

practicalities

Simple hygiene can play a helpful role in managing infectious conjunctivitis.

- Keep face cloths and towels clean.

- Never share cosmetic brushes. Wash them regularly with a gentle detergent, rinsing well to remove any soapy residue.

- Always wash your hands before and after touching your eyes.

- Use separate cotton wool pads for cleaning any crustiness from each eyelid and throw them away afterwards.

homeopathy

Aconite Use this to ease any rapidly developing symptoms that appear after exposure to dry, cold winds. In this case, the eyes feel dry and gritty, and the eyelids often feel and look quite swollen.

Belladonna This is helpful if the eyes feel hot and burning, the whites are unusually bloodshot, and the symptoms have appeared very quickly. When this remedy is needed, the eyes are a lot more sensitive to light, so you may feel like half-closing them.

Pulsatilla This remedy is better for conjunctivitis that develops in the late stages of a catarrhal cold and is ideal when the eyelashes are stuck together by a yellow crust on waking. It also produces a characteristic sensation of something covering the eye, which may make you want to rub it.

Apis Use this to soothe conjunctivitis that becomes more uncomfortable in warm surroundings. Your eyelids may look puffy and swollen, with a pinkish tinge and you may be very reluctant to have your eyes covered because of their sensitivity.

western herbalism

Bathe your eyes with this soothing lotion to ease the soreness and itching of mild conjunctitvitis.

Dilute 4 drops of Euphrasia tincture in 140 ml (5 fl oz) of cooled, boiled water.

styes

These unpleasant swellings tend to develop whenever the small glands at the roots of the eyelashes becoming infected and inflamed. As a result, pus starts to form, sometimes in considerable amounts. The average stye lasts for approximately 7 days, after which it should clear up. The appearance of a stye can vary from a small, raised swelling to a large, puffy, angry-looking lump.

common symptoms

- **Discomfort at the base of one eyelash**
- **Formation of an abscess with a yellow head**
- **Some swelling of the affected eyelid**

conventional treatments

The odd stye does not require any conventional treatment, but if you find they are occurring regularly, a course of antibiotics may be necessary to clear up the infection. While styes are not a major concern in themselves, recurrent problems can suggest that you may be generally run down.

complementary treatments

Any of the self-help measures listed below may be used in the short-term to speed up the healing process and relieve some of the discomfort caused by a stye. As with blepharitis (see page 100), if styes occur on a regular basis, you should consult an alternative or complementary therapist, who will attempt to eradicate the underlying cause of the problem.

homeopathy

Belladonna Use this to soothe a stye that forms suddenly, with pronounced symptoms. The affected area of the eyelid may be hot to the touch and very red, and the eye may feel very dry and gritty.

Apis This is better for styes that result in a very puffy eyelid that looks rosy-pink and water-logged. The symptoms, unlike those relieved by Belladonna, include the production of a lot of tears in the affected eye, which burn and sting. The application of cool compresses brings temporary relief, while warmth increases the discomfort.

Hepar sulphuris calcareum (Hepar sulph.) This is best for large, swollen styes that produce a lot of yellowish pus. Exposure to draughts of cold air causes much distress, triggering localized, sharp, splinter-type pains. Warm bathing will temporarily ease general discomfort around the eyelid.

Pulsatilla This remedy is good for styes of lower eyelids, especially if they have reached the stage where the eyelids are stuck together by a yellow crust in morning. The stye is likely to be very itchy, leading to a constant urge to rub the eyes. Warmth usually increases the discomfort in the eyelid.

nutritional approaches

Too much sugar encourages the establishment of bacterial and fungal infections so you should cut your sugar intake if styes are becoming a regular feature. The most common sources of white, refined sugar are biscuits, cakes, fizzy drinks, chocolate and ice cream.

naturopathy

Include regular helpings of garlic in your diet or take a course of garlic tablets. Garlic is very helpful because of its blood-purifying, anti-viral and antibiotic properties.

western herbalism

• Apply a warm compress of diluted Calendula tincture (1 part tincture to 10 parts of cooled, boiled water). This can be immensely soothing to a stye that is at the early, inflamed stage. Because of its natural healing properties, Calendula is also an excellent choice for discouraging infection.

• If stye formation is accompanied by a general feeling of being under par, take a short course of Echinacea until the problem clears up. Note that taking this on a long-term basis appears to be counterproductive.

blepharitis

People who suffer from eczema or dandruff are particularly susceptible to blepharitis and some cosmetics may act as trigger. This irritating condition arises when the rims of the eyelids become infected and inflamed, leading to sore, itchy, scaly-looking eyelids. If the skin becomes very flaky, particles of skin can enter the eye and trigger further infection, such as conjunctivitis.

common symptoms

- **Eyelid rims become swollen, red, scaly and itchy**
- **Crusting of the eyelids**
- **Development of small ulcers on the eyelid rims, sometimes with loss of eyelashes**

conventional treatments

Doctors usually prescribe antibiotic and steroid preparations which you apply to the rims of the eyelids.

complementary treatments

Since blepharitis is a chronic problem, it is best to consult an experienced practitioner if treatment is to be most successful. In the meantime, any of the following self-help measures may relieve some of the symptoms in the short term.

homeopathy

Graphites This may ease classic blepharitis symptoms, such as dry, scaly, red eyelids with a tendency to in-growing lashes, especially if there are patches of eczema on the scalp and eyelids, and a tendency for the eyelids to crack and become sore.

naturopathy

Gently bathe the edges of the eyelids with a cottonwool bud soaked in a warm, weak solution of salt and water. This should soothe the irritated skin in the short term. If this causes any stinging or discomfort, add more water to the solution or try one of the herbal solutions listed below.

western herbalism

Bathe the inflamed irritated skin at the eyelid rims with diluted Calendula tincture. Dilute 1 part of tincture in 10 parts of cooled, boiled water. If you find this soothing, applying a tiny amount of Calendula cream to the area above the lid margins may help preserve the effect.

bloodshot eyes

The condition can be triggered by any of the factors listed below. It's wise to treat any marked symptoms of bloodshot eyes with respect, since they can sometimes be indicative of a more serious problem. Should severe pain, redness and watering occur (especially if only in one eye), it's important to seek prompt medical advice.

common triggers

- **Too many late nights**
- **Eye strain resulting from reading in poor light or long spells at a computer screen**
- **An eye infection, such as conjunctivitis**
- **A reaction to contact lenses or a cosmetic product**

conventional treatments

Unless there is an underlying infection, these tend to involve the use of soothing eye drops and basic advice on positive lifestyle changes, such as getting regular early nights, ensuring that you have adequate lighting at work, and having your eyes checked by an optician in order to rectify any eye strain problems.

complementary treatments

If there is no underling infection, a one-off episode of bloodshot eyes may be soothed by any of the following treatments.

naturopathy

- Avoid any eye drops that claim to make the whites of the eyes sparkle. These work by temporarily narrowing the blood vessels in the eyes. When the effects wear off, the whites of the eyes will look even redder than before.
- Instead, try a reviving technique called 'palming,' which can put the sparkle back in tired, red eyes without any side-effects. Gently rest the cupped palms of both hands over your closed eyes while taking deep breaths to relax the body. Keep the palms in this position for approximately 5 minutes for a relaxing, restorative treat.

western herbalism

- To restore their sparkle, bathe tired, strained eyes with this soothing lotion.

Add 4 drops of Euphrasia tincture to 140 ml (5 fl oz) of cooled, boiled water.

- Cooled infusions of soothing herbal teas, such as chamomile or elderflower, can feel incredibly reviving to red, tired eyes. Soak a couple of cottonwool pads in the infusion and place them lightly over your closed eyes for a few minutes.

spots and acne

At times of hormonal change, women can be dismayed to find themselves breaking out in spots. Acne is most likely to emerge at puberty, but can also occur at menopause. Remember that a tendency to develop spots can be a barometer of health as well as just a cosmetic nuisance. As a result, you may need to change aspects of your lifestyle to regain a healthy balance, rather than relying on special creams and washes.

times of hormonal change

- **Adolescence**
- **Before and after periods**
- **Pregnancy**
- **Menopause**

common triggers

- **A high-stress lifestyle**
- **Eating a lot of convenience foods, which contain fat and sugar, plus colourings and preservatives**
- **Too little exercise**
- **Lack of good-quality sleep**
- **Use of abrasive, heavy-duty cleansers or exfoliators**
- **Drinking too little water**
- **Chronic constipation**
- **Progesterone-dominant contraceptives such as the mini-pill, progesterone implants or injections**

conventional treatments

Treatment of acne often involves the long-term use of low-dose antibiotics, coupled with antiseptic lotions and washes designed to dry out the spots quickly. A doctor may prescribe one of the retinoid drugs, which dramatically reduce oil production in the skin, but sometimes have off-putting side-effects.

complementary treatments

Any of the following self-help treatments may be used to gently but effectively improve overall skin texture. Do bear in mind that poor-quality skin can be indicative of a more deep-seated imbalance in the system. If this is the case, it will be helpful to tackle the problem from inside (by improving overall health and vitality), rather than concentrating only on surface measures to manage the problem.

aromatherapy

Apply the following blend after cleansing and before taking a bath or shower (to encourage effective penetration). Gently wipe off any residue with a clean cottonwool pad after half an hour.

Add 1 drop each of patchouli and frankincense and 2 drops of lavender essential oil to 25 ml of jojoba carrier oil.

homeopathy

Belladonna A few doses are taken at the early inflamed stage encourages the odd, isolated spot to heal, or may push things on to the stage where the spot develops a pus-filled head.

Hepar sulphuris calcareum (Hepar sulph.) This quickly deals with any spots that have developed a pus-filled head if a few doses are taken at this stage.

Silicea terra (Silica) A couple of doses taken once the spot has broken and the final stage of healing is underway will discourage long-lasting scar formation.

nutritional approaches

• Vitamin C is vitally important in preserving healthy skin tone and texture and fighting infection, but is easily destroyed during food preparation and cooking. Take a supplement, especially during the winter when you may not eat enough fresh fruit and vegetables. If you have an outbreak of spots, take 500 mg of a slow-release formula of vitamin C every day for a week.

• Avoid fatty, greasy and sugary foods and increase your intake of fresh fruit and vegetables.

• Drink five or six glasses of filtered or still mineral water each day. Keeping up your fluid intake assists the detoxifying and eliminatory processes of the kidneys and bowel.

naturopathy

For a cleansing face mask, mix oatmeal and natural yoghurt to a thick paste. Spread over the affected area and allow it to dry before gently rinsing off.

western herbalism

• To treat oily skin, make a herbal cleansing serum by blending equal portions of rose or elderflower water with fresh lemon juice. If your skin is sensitive as well as oily, carry out a patch test on a tiny area first.

• Apply the following soothing, healing lotion to any skin blemishes. Marigold has healing, antiseptic properties, while wheatgerm oil encourages scarred tissues to heal.

Add 2 tablespoonful of dried, powdered marigold petals to 4 tablespoonful of warmed wheatgerm oil. Strain off the liquid and store it in a stoppered bottle.

puffy eyelids

Temporary puffiness and mild swelling around the eyes are usually triggered by over-indulgence. Caused by accumulation of fluid in the tissues, it is aggravated by rubbing. Puffy eyes can also be hyper-sensitive or allergic reactions (such as hay fever). If this is the case, you will benefit from some professional complementary treatment.

common triggers

- **Too little sleep**
- **Too much partying**
- **An over-taxed liver that has had to deal with too much alcohol**
- **Crying**
- **An underactive thyroid gland**

conventional treatments

If your eyes are also red, itchy, and/or sore, consult your doctor or optician. You may have conjunctivitis (see pages 96–97), in which case soothing, antibiotic drops or ointment should clear up the condition very quickly.

complementary treatments

Any of the following self-help measures can calm and soothe puffy eyes.

ayurveda

Soak two cottonwool pads in cool milk (ideally from the refrigerator) and apply to the area around the eyes each morning.

nutritional approaches

Tired-looking eyes suggest that the kidneys are being overworked. Avoid foods that are regarded as acid-forming, such as white rice or refined (white) grains, convenience foods and caffeinated drinks like coffee, tea and colas. Drink plenty of filtered water to flush out the kidneys and eat alkaline-forming fruit and vegetables.

naturopathy

Place two thin slices of cucumber on each closed eye and relax for 5 minutes.

western herbalism

- Drink dandelion tea to encourage the body to flush away excess fluid, which can aggravate a tendency to puffiness around the eyes.

- If you feel in need of a general detox, take a supplement of milk thistle, which has a reputation for aiding detoxification.

- Soak cottonwool pads in the following diluted Euphrasia tincture, wring them out and placed them gently over each closed eye while you rest for 10 minutes.

warts and veruccas

Warts are similar to cold sores in being triggered by the presence of a virus in the body. The areas most commonly affected include the hands and feet (where they become flattened and are known as veruccas). Since warts are due to a virus in the system, it will be helpful to seek ways of supporting immune system functioning if the problem is to be dealt with effectively.

common symptoms

- **A raised area of skin a few millimetres across**
- **This area has a rough surface**
- **Tiny black dots, caused by clotted blood in the capillaries, may be visible in the centre**

conventional treatments

Treatment tends to focus on removing the warts or veruccas by freezing them with chemicals, such as liquid nitrogen, or burning them, and scraping them off under local anaesthetic. Over-the-counter creams contain salicylic acid, which destroys the thick skin. This may take months but the careful use of an emery board may speed up the process.

complementary treatments

For well-established or severe problems, consult a trained practitioner, who will try to tackle the problem on two levels. Treatment is usually aimed at expelling the problem from within, by removing the imbalance in the system that is causing the warts. Your practitioner may also suggest applying a topical preparation, such as Thuja tincture (see right). For the odd tiny wart or verucca, the following self-help measures may be useful.

naturopathy

- Take supplements of vitamins A, C and E, which are all anti-oxidants with a good reputation for supporting an effective and balanced immune system.

- Take a powdered garlic supplement with a high allicin content to clear up a wart that is already healing.

western herbalism

Diluted Thuja tincture can be applied to the wart to encourage it to shrink.

Dissolve 1 teaspoonful of Thuja tincture in a cup of water, and dab the solution on the wart for 10 days.

dandruff

This irritating condition may be triggered by the presence of a fungus, but this is considered to be debatable in some medical circles. This is present in everyone, but some people over-react to it. If you have an underlying tendency to psoriasis, you may constantly feel like giving your scalp a good scratch. Apart from the white scales that fall onto the shoulders, making wearing dark clothes quite impractical, dandruff can also make the hair look dull and lifeless.

common symptoms

- **Build-up of dead skin cells on the scalp**
- **Dryness and flaking of the scalp**

conventional treatments

Treatment tends to concentrate on the use of shampoos and/or lotions designed to lift and remove the dry scales. For serious cases, an anti-fungal shampoo may be advisable. Unfortunately, all these can sometimes aggravate the condition by making the scalp even drier.

complementary treatments

In mild cases, the following can be of help in the short term. However, well-established skin problems tend to be an indication of a more deep-seated imbalance in the system, so you may need professional help to eradicate the problem. A complementary practitioner would aim (as they always do regardless of the medical condition or problem) to stimulate a greater sense of balance within the system as a whole. Treatment, of course needs to be individualized for the most positive reaction to emerge.

aromatherapy

Massage your scalp with the following blend of essential oils.

Add 2–3 drops of cedarwood, lavender and rosemary essential oils to a small saucerful of carrier oil.

naturopathy

If dandruff is a problem, take care to rinse out all traces of shampoo when washing your hair. Any build-up of residue may cause further problems of skin dryness and making the hair look dull and lifeless.

western herbalism

Use a scalp-conditioning infusion of nettles, rosemary and sage as a rinse after hair washing. Alternatively, use a commercial natural shampoo containing these herbs.

dry skin

The skin is normally kept in good condition by oily glandular secretions and moisture. If these are removed, taut, dry patches of flaking skin may appear, especially if the skin is sensitive. It is a particular problem during the winter, due to the extremes of weather and long periods in centrally heated surroundings. However comforting central heating may be, it has a significantly drying effect on the skin and mucous membranes.

common triggers

- **Contact with detergents or strong soaps, which remove the natural oil**
- **Exposure to strong sunlight or harsh, drying winds**
- **Age – the skin glands become less efficient over time**
- **Central heating**
- **Smoking**

conventional treatments

These revolve around ways of putting moisture back into the skin, such as using aqueous cream as a moisturizer or, in very severe cases (especially where dry skin is combined with a tendency to eczema), washing with an emulsifying cream rather than soap.

complementary treatments

Any of the following can provide temporary relief from the discomfort of recent small patches of dry skin.

naturopathy

- Avoid using harsh, detergent-based skin-care products. Also avoid highly perfumed items if your skin tends to be sensitive as well as dry, in order to avoid aggravating this tendency.

- Use rosewater, which is gentle on the skin, rather than alcohol-based toners, which can aggravate any tendency to dryness.

- Choose skin-care products containing ingredients such as evening primrose oil, cucumber, lavender and chamomile, which have a reputation for being 'friendly' to dry, sensitive skin.

- Remember the important therapeutic effects of water. Drink at least six large glasses of filtered or still mineral water a day. Place a bowl of water beside every radiator at home and at work to combat the drying effect of central heating.

western herbalism

For small outbreaks of cracked, dry skin (for instance, at the corners of the mouth), apply Calendula cream at regular intervals during the day. Apart from being an excellent lightweight moisturizer, it also encourages the speedy healing of damaged skin.

eczema

Eczema is caused by an over-reaction of the skin, sometimes to an irritant, sometimes not. It is not the same as dermatitis, which is clearly due to an irritant. It often occurs in people with a heightened immune system (atopic eczema) or may be triggered by contact with an irritant substance (contact eczema). Symptoms of eczema, which vary greatly in their range and severity, are listed below.

common symptoms

- **Redness and inflammation of the skin**
- **Severe itching that can be so severe that the skin is broken through scratching**
- **Dryness and flaking of affected areas or weepy, crusty patches**

conventional treatments

Steroid creams tend to be the first line of treatment for eczema in children and adults. Where itching is especially severe, a doctor may prescribe antihistamines as well. Wet wrapping may be applied to severly affected areas.

complementary treatments

Any of the following can be used to ease the irritation, itching and soreness of a minor patch of eczema. However, if the condition is well-established and/or widespread, you should consult a trained complementary therapist who will aim to treat the underlying cause of the condition.

homeopathy

Rhus toxicodendron (Rhus tox.) This should soothe patches of intensely itchy skin that are maddening at night, especially if the patches start as small, itchy blisters that become crusty and weepy after scratching. The affected skin is usually painfully sensitive to cold air and better in warm, dry weather.

Arsenicum album This remedy is better for dry, rough, burning skin that alternates with asthma, especially if symptoms worsen when you are anxious and stressed. Surprisingly, the burning sensation is usually eased by a warm bath.

Graphites This may ease weeping eczema in the folds of skin (for instance, behind the ears or at the corners of the mouth). It is best suited to eczema that produces a honey-coloured fluid which dries to a hard crust, especially where symptoms intensify before and after a period.

nutritional approaches

Avoid foods that have a reputation for aggravating eczema, such as wheat, convenience foods that contain colourings, additives and preservatives, potatoes, tomatoes, aubergines and green peppers, dairy foods and eggs, and sugar.

naturopathy

• When using detergents, choose brands specially formulated for people with allergic or sensitive skins. Most importantly, always rinse items thoroughly to remove any detergent residue.

• If you have contact eczema, always wear thin cotton gloves when working in the kitchen. If you are sensitive to rubber, try another type of waterproof glove or wear cotton gloves beneath. Take particular care when chopping items that have a reputation for sparking off an allergic response, such as potatoes, tomatoes or citrus fruits.

• Keep areas of sensitive, dry or itchy skin well moisturized, especially in cold, windy weather, or after bathing or showering. Apply liberal amounts of emulsifying or aqueous cream after bathing. Remember that dry, taut skin will become itchy more quickly than soft, moisturized skin.

• An oatmeal bath may soothe and nourish dry, irritated skin. Add a couple of generous tablespoonsful of oatmeal to a muslin bag and suspend this beneath the hot tap as you run your bath.

western herbalism

• Apply this soothing compress of Calendula to sore, itchy skin.

Add 1 teaspoonful of Calendula lotion to a glass of boiled, cooled water.

• If this is soothing, prolong the effect by applying Calendula cream or ointment at regular intervals. The cream is lightly moisturizing and naturally antiseptic, while the ointment is more suited to very parched, dry skin (provided the user can tolerate lanolin).

psoriasis

This is one of the many conditions associated with high or poorly managed stress levels and it commonly becomes worse during, or following, periods of high tension. Symptoms may also become more obvious after a throat infection, or after a course of drugs for rheumatoid arthritis or malaria. They can also vary from small, mild outbreaks to a skin eruption that causes a great deal of distress and discomfort.

common symptoms

- **Large, oval patches of thickened, scaly, blistering skin that cover the elbows, knees and scalp**
- **Affected areas may be intensely itchy**
- **In severe cases, the nails thicken so that they are forced to grow away from the nail bed**
- **A form of arthritis commonly affecting the joints of the hips, sacro-illiac joints, fingers and feet**

conventional treatments

These tend to rely on creams, lotions and shampoos aimed at easing itching and scaling. Unfortunately some of these are unpleasant to use because of their messy texture and unattractive smell. If symptoms do not respond to this avenue of treatment, ultra-violet light treatment (PUVA) may be an option.

complementary treatments

As with eczema, because psoriasis tends to be well-established and chronic, it is best to consult an experienced practitioner. Chinese herbalism has an especially impressive track record for the successful treatment of skin conditions. However, some of the following self-help strategies may give temporary relief.

homeopathy

Calcarea carbonica (Calc. carb.) This may improve pale, unhealthy skin that has a tendency to chap, dry out and crack easily. The overall picture tends to be one of sluggishness, with skin feeling cold and clammy to the touch and showing a general tendency to slow healing.

Lycopodium Dry, raw-feeling, sensitive skin that becomes much worse during or following an anxious or stressful time may be eased by this remedy. It is indicated where the scalp is especially affected and the skin on the hands and soles of the feet is especially dry and cracked.

nutritional approaches

• Avoid foods that have a negative reputation with regard to skin problems, such as red meat, animal fats and sugar. Items that appear to have a beneficial effect include whole grains, pulses, vegetables (avoiding potatoes and tomatoes) and fruit (but not citrus fruit).

• Eat foods that are rich in essential fatty acids, such as herrings, mackerel and salmon, which appear to have a beneficial effect on psoriasis. Evening primrose oil is another good source of fatty acids.

naturopathy

• Exposure to sunshine may improve some cases of psoriasis. However, be sure to use protective creams, cover any delicate areas of skin and avoid going out when the sun's rays are at their strongest (noon until late afternoon).

• Bathing in a solution of sea salts or Dead Sea salts can also benefit dry, flaky skin. Nevertheless, it is advisable to do a patch test first: bathe a small area of skin in a solution of sea salts on three or four nights to see how it responds. If all is well, you can then use the salts in the bath, following the manufacturer's instructions.

western herbalism

Chickweed cream can soothe patches of dry, itchy, cracked skin. Use an infusion to rinse the hair after washing to ease an itchy, scaly scalp.

active therapies

If stress management is an issue, investigate ways of relaxing more effectively. Options to consider may include meditation, guided relaxation exercises, autogenic training and/or progressive muscular relaxation.

cold sores

Most people have a virus known as herpes simplex in their bodies. This virus tends to remain dormant when immune systems are working well. However, stress, a nasty cold or too much time in strong sunlight may trigger the formation of cold sores, which is why they are regarded as a sign of being generally 'run down'. It therefore makes sense to concentrate on boosting the immune system to discourage their appearance.

common symptoms

- **An itching and/or tingling sensation of the affected area (such as the around the lips or under the nose)**
- **A painful blister may form as the discomfort gathers momentum**
- **Once the blister bursts, it takes on the characteristic crusty appearance of a cold sore**

conventional treatments

The application of an anti-viral preparation to the cold sores can minimize the severity of the outbreak if you catch it early enough. It's generally thought that these preparations work most effectively when used at the very first sign of a problem. So, for the best results to have a chance to emerge, take action at the very first twinge or tingle.

complementary treatments

As with any other skin condition, it is best to consult a trained practitioner in order to successfully eradicate the problem from within. However, some of the following self-help measures can be used as a damage limitation exercise, minimizing the pain of the cold sore and speeding up the healing process.

practicalities

• The virus that causes cold sores can be carried on a toothbrush. Therefore, once the cold sore reaches the blister stage, throw away your current toothbrush and buy a new one to prevent any re-infection.

• Avoid kissing anyone and also avoid oral sex, even if the cold sore is only at the tingling stage and has not yet made a full appearance.

• If you have a history of cold sores, invest in an ultra-violet lip-block and use it whenever you go out in sunny, windy weather. This is also a good habit to adopt if you go skiing at high altitudes, where the reflection of bright sunlight on snow can be especially harsh.

aromatherapy

Add 2 drops of lavender oil to a clean cottonwool bud and dab on the affected area three or four times a day.

homeopathy

Natrum muriaticum (Natrum mur.) This is indicated where there is a tendency to cold sores after exposure to bright sunlight or very windy weather. Sores especially affect the mouth and lips, and the lips feel dry and tend to crack easily (especially in the middle).

Rhus toxicodendron (Rhus tox.) This is better for cold sores that feel numb or tingly and tend to affect the mouth and lips, especially if the lips get very dry and tend to crack easily in the corners.

nutritional approaches

If a cold sore is large, especially sensitive and extends from the lip into the inner part of the mouth, avoid contact with foods that cause stinging or smarting, such as salty snacks, citrus fruits and drinks containing lemon juice.

naturopathy

• Apply aloe vera gel to soothe and cool a painful cold sore.

• Dab a cold sore from time to time with a small amount of witch hazel. This can also encourage a cold sore to dry up when it has reached at the blister stage.

western herbalism

Apply the following to the cold sore as a speedy and effective way of boosting the healing process and providing temporary relief of pain and discomfort.

Dilute 1 part Hypericum tincture to 10 parts of cooled, boiled water and apply the solution on a cottonwool pad.

brittle nails

The overall condition of your skin, hair and nails can reveal a great deal about your basic level of health. Clear skin, shining hair and strong nails suggest that you are on good form, while poor skin tone and colour, dull hair, and nails that break easily all suggest less than optimum health. Apart from poor nutrition or recovery from a phase of severe ill health, there are other factors that can lead to poor-quality, brittle nails.

habits to avoid

- Constantly washing hands in strong detergents
- Careless rinsing and drying of hands
- Not paying enough attention to moisturizing hands and nails
- Over-use of nail polish, because nail-polish remover can have a generally drying effect on the nails
- Fungal infections, which may lead to overgrowth and weakness of the nail

conventional treatments

Skin problems such as psoriasis (see pages 110–111) can cause brittleness and discolouration of the nails.

complementary treatments

Breaking bad habits and paying attention to the condition of your nails may be sufficient. However, if the problem persists, you should consider professional complementary medical support, such as nutritional therapy.

practicalities

• Massage the hands regularly, paying particular attention to the cuticles, which play a vital role in nail nourishment. Never cut the cuticles, but push them back gently when they are damp. After washing, apply a moisturizing hand cream, working it into the cuticles.

• Make a point of massaging a nourishing oil into the nails each night before sleep. Choose a specially formulated nail oil or sweet almond oil, which is light and easily absorbed.

• Regular application of nail strengthener (but not one that includes formaldehyde) may benefit nails that are prone to occasional chipping and flaking but are otherwise in good health.

• To encourage maximum nail strength, file the nails regularly using an emery board, working in one direction only. This is important because friction tends to weaken the fabric of the nails.

nutritional approaches

• Strong nails thrive on a well-balanced diet that provides all basic nutrients. Calcium (found in dairy foods and green leafy vegetables, nuts, wholegrains and pulses) is particularly valuable. Balance calcium intake with magnesium and vitamin D to aid absorption.

hair loss

As we get older, there is a natural tendency for hair to become thinner. This is related to the hair follicles becoming less efficient at holding on to the hairs that they contain. Certain lifestyle factors, hormonal imbalances or medical problems, such as thyroid imbalance or a condition called alopecia, may also contribute to significant hair loss.

common triggers

• **Stress or shock**

• **Poor diet**

• **Hormonal changes (due to pregnancy or menopause)**

• **Chemical damage**

conventional treatments

If hair loss is due to alopecia, doctors usually recommend stress management techniques as this condition is known to be stress related. Cases of extensive hair loss may be referred to a specialist, who may advise steroid injections into the scalp to stimulate regrowth.

complementary treatments

Treatments are most likely to focus on underlying stress factors, such as poor diet, too little sleep or poor recovery after a distressing or traumatic event. If symptoms are very generalized and mild, the following advice may be helpful.

practicalities

Massage the scalp regularly to stimulate blood flow to the hair follicles and help mild hair loss. Use the tips of the fingers to make small circular movements from the forehead to the nape of the neck until you have covered the entire scalp.

nutritional approaches

• A healthy diet will pay huge dividends, since hair follicles depend on a balanced supply of basic nutrients in order to develop a strong, resilient, shiny strand of hair. Millet is thought to be one of the most effective hair-boosters because it provides a substantial number of the essential amino acids needed by the hair to stay in good condition.

• Millet also contains the all-important vitamin B complex. The nutrients of the B complex have a particularly powerful dual role to play because they encourage the growth of healthy hair as well as supporting the nervous system at times of stress. A vitamin B supplement can also be taken, but it is important to take a complex formula, rather than any of the B vitamins in isolation as this can cause neurological symptoms.

boils

A tendency to recurrent boils is traditionally associated with being run down – any recurring skin condition that shows signs of poor healing is a sign that the body's defences are at a low ebb. Boils are infections of the hair shafts, resulting from bacteria entering through small nicks or abrasions in the skin. The emergence of one or several boils at once may be a sign of underlying problems, such as a poor diet or diabetes.

common symptoms

- **Heat, redness and swelling of the affected area**
- **Throbbing**
- **Pus-formation**

conventional treatments

One large boil, or a group of boils clustered together (collectively called a carbuncle), may require antibiotic treatment or it may be necessary to lance them. Your doctor may prescribe an antiseptic or antibiotic cream for a small boil or oral antibiotics if the boil is larger than 1 cm (½ in) across.

complementary treatments

Treatments are likely to concentrate on boosting the body's natural defences, as well as using natural topical preparations to speed up the healing process and discourage scarring.

aromatherapy

Apply 1 drop of niaouli to a clean cottonwool bud and dab gently on the surface of the boil to encourage speedy healing. This minor essential oil has an excellent reputation for gently but effectively encouraging the elimination of bacterial and viral infections.

homeopathy

Belladonna Use this during the first stage of inflammation, when there is a lot of heat in the area of the boil and an obvious bright redness of the skin.

Hepar sulphuris calcareum (Hepar sulph.) This remedy will quickly resolve the situation once the boil has moved on to the pus formation stage after a few doses, especially if the discharge tends to be thick and yellow.

Silicea terra (Silica) This remedy will help to avoid scarring when taken during the last stage of healing and is indicated for thin, watery discharges.

naturopathy

• Drink six large glasses of filtered tap or mineral water each day in order to help the kidneys flush out toxins effectively from the body. In this way you will avoid any low-level dehydration, which has an adverse effect on skin quality in general.

• Avoid 'quick-fix' or junk foods, since these invariably have an adverse effect on the skin. Instead, choose good-quality wholefoods, such as fresh fruit, vegetables, pulses, wholegrains (such as brown rice) and small amounts of fish and organic poultry. Also avoid spicy, fatty or sweetened foods that are especially rich in refined white sugar.

• Smoking and alcohol are other lifestyle factors that have an adverse effect on skin tone and quality. If your skin shows genuine signs of being unhealthy, it may be helpful to take a course of vitamin C for the duration of the outbreak. Take a slow-release capsule of 500 mg morning and evening.

• Apply a warm compress to soothe a boil when it is at the 'drawing' stage and especially painful. This need involve nothing more complicated than a clean face cloth, wrung out after soaking in warm water.

western herbalism

• Once a boil has burst or been lanced by a doctor or nurse, apply Calendula cream to encourage fast healing of tissue and lessen the risk of infection.

• Take a course of Echinacea internally to support the immune system while it is fighting infection.

cellulite

Cellulite (bumpy skin with an 'orange peel' appearance) on thighs, belly, buttocks or upper arms is far more common in women than men. It is caused by the accumulation of fat in the fat cells and loss of tone in the tissue that supports them. Several complementary therapies regard a significant amount of cellulite as a sign of the system being overloaded with toxins, possibly due to sluggish movement of the lymphatic fluid and poor diet.

common triggers

- The enlargement of female fat cells at puberty in response to increased oestrogen
- The thickening of connective tissue and thinning and loss of elasticity of surface skin as women grow older. Dimples appear as the skin becomes less resistant to the bulging fat chambers beneath
- Increased water retention due to oral contraceptives which applies pressure on the surface skin layers
- Excess weight – enlarged fat cells upset circulation, contributing to the appearance of cellulite
- Poor diet – especially the consumption of too many fatty acids

conventional treatments

Conventional medicine tends to be fairly dismissive of cellulite, often regarding it as no more than an undesirable consequence of being overweight. This is a rather controversial area because, although cellulite can be exacerbated by overweight, many women of ideal weight still have noticeable signs of cellulite on their bodies.

complementary treatments

Many complementary therapists regard the texture, tone and appearance of the skin as being indicative of inner health, and the existence of cellulite is no exception. Instead of concentrating solely on dealing with areas of cellulite from without, many of the complementary medical strategies for cellulite-busting listed below attempt to banish the problem from within.

aromatherapy

In addition to the measures above, using a special cellulite-removing blend of massage cream or oil can speed up progress. The massaging movement alone can stimulate sluggish circulation of the lymphatic fluid, and the active ingredients of the essential oils help to improve skin tone and texture.

nutritional approaches

• Since the presence of cellulite has been linked to a general state of sluggishness and toxic overload, concentrate on eliminating as many junk foods as possible from your diet. Foods to avoid include coffee, alcohol, foods high in saturated fat (such as full-fat cheese, cream and red meat), convenience foods, and any items containing large amounts of white sugar (including the 'hidden' sugars in sauces and fizzy drinks).

• Drink eight large glasses of water a day to aid efficient detoxification. Avoid too much carbonated water, which can lead to abdominal bloating.

naturopathy

• Regular dry-skin body-brushing with a natural bristle brush is considered an effective way of stimulating the lymphatic circulation. This depends on muscular contractions of the arms and legs rather than having a pump, like the heart.

Before your daily shower or bath, make long, sweeping strokes over your body using a long-handled, natural bristle brush. Move up your body, from feet to hips and belly, using long, firm strokes. Then move up the arms in the same way, paying special attention to the inside of the upper arms where skin can easily become bumpy and slack.

• Regular exercise also stimulates the lymphatic circulation and is considered a must if you want to keep cellulite at bay and improve the tone and appearance of your skin.

• Avoid long soaking in a very hot bath, or going on yo-yo diets that result in alternating periods of significant weight loss and weight gain. These can make you more vulnerable to cellulite and also adversely affect skin tone in general.

foot health

It is amazing how much we take our feet for granted. We walk on them all day, stand for hours and often subject them to punishing footwear in the name of style and fashion. Despite this harsh treatment, we tend to ignore any minor foot problems. In fairness, this is hardly surprising, since our feet are under cover for a large part of the year and, unless a problem is painful, we tend to put off taking action until another day.

common problems

- **Veruccas**
- **Sweaty feet**
- **Athlete's foot**
- **Corns and calluses**
- **In-growing toenails**

conventional treatments

Treatments usually involve anti-fungal type medication for athlete's foot or mechanical removal of veruccas (see Warts and verrucas, page 105) to make the feet more comfortable in the long run. Visits to a chiropodist or podiatrist, who both specialize in issues of foot health, will keep your feet in good general condition.

complementary treatments

Any of the following treatments can provide natural, additional support in dealing with common foot problems.

practicalities

• Visit your chiropodist on a regular basis so that any problems can be dealt with before they become severe.

• Remove rough skin by using an exfoliating preparation, concentrating on rough areas of skin on the sole and heel, before massaging your feet with a moisturizing cream or cooling gel.

• Avoid in-growing toenails by clipping your toenails as straight across as possible, in line with the tops of the toes. Never cut a curve into the side of the toenail because this can encourage the nail to grow inwards.

• Make sure that the shoes you are wearing give adequate, comfortable support to your feet, without cramping your toes. Check with your chiropodist if necessary.

• To treat corns and calluses, gently but firmly rub the area of hardened skin with a pumice stone exfoliating pad while bathing.

• For hard corns, apply a few drops of wheatgerm oil to the affected area before bed in order to soften the skin.

• Dry thoroughly between the toes after bathing to avoid any friction occurring and apply witch hazel twice daily. This discourages the build-up of sweat in these warm areas.

aromatherapy

• If you have sweaty feet, bathe your feet every day in this naturally deodorizing foot bath to keep your feet fresh. Soak your feet for approximately 5 minutes before drying them thoroughly, particularly between the toes.

Add 3 drops of lavender and 3 drops of sage essential oils to 1.5 litres (just over 3 pints) of comfortably warm water.

• To treat athlete's foot, apply the following antifungal blend twice a day to affected areas until it disappears.

Add 15 drops of lavender and 15 drops of myrrh essential oil to 30 ml (1 fl oz) of carrier oil.

nutritional approaches

Athlete's foot and fungal infections in general can be discouraged by eating a bowl of natural, live yoghurt each day, because of its natural probiotic content. Natural yoghurt containing *Lactobacillus acidophilus* is thought to have a beneficial effect by helping to restore the natural balance of micro-organisms in the gut.

naturopathy

• If you have sweaty feet, avoid wearing shoes made from synthetic materials, such as plastic, for any length of time because this can make the feet sweat more. Also avoid wearing the same pair of shoes for two consecutive days. It also helps to spend as much time as possible with bare feet, in order to allow the skin of the feet to breathe.

• Discourage any problems with infection between the toes by regular application of a naturally antiseptic cream containing propolis. This can also encourage any areas of damaged skin to heal quickly and well.

sore throats and tonsillitis

Whenever you have a severe sore throat, it helps to remember that the tonsils are our first line of defence. Inflamed and painful tonsils are a sign that they are busily fighting infection. Apart from infection, other triggers of a sore throat include talking for a long time or being in a smoky atmosphere. The symptoms of tonsillitis are quite easy to spot and can include any combination of those listed below.

common symptoms

- **High temperature**
- **Headaches**
- **Shivers and aching all over the body**
- **Extreme pain and swelling in the throat, causing difficulty in swallowing**
- **Vomiting**
- **Foul breath with a dreadful taste in the mouth**
- **Swollen, painful glands**
- **A general sense of malaise and feeling very unwell**

conventional treatments

For simple sore throats, the general advice is likely to include taking lots of fluid, gargling with a painkiller and sucking on throat lozenges that contain a short-acting local anaesthetic. A bout of tonsillitis will need antibiotic treatment in order to deal with the infection as quickly as possible.

complementary treatments

Any combination of the self-help measures suggested below will significantly ease a simple sore throat. However, for a bout of tonsillitis, it is worth considering some additional complementary medical support to accompany the antibiotic treatment.

practicalities

• Whenever possible, avoid anything that is likely to put extra strain on your throat and voice, such as not over-straining the voice. You should also avoid smoking or socializing in smoky surroundings, and give the throat and voice a chance to rest and relax.

• Sucking throat pastilles designed to provide lubrication can help to relieve the dry sensation that is often part and parcel of a sore throat.

aromatherapy

Make this soothing massage blend and massage it gently into the area of the throat three times a day.

Add 3 drops of eucalyptus and tea tree essential oils to 2 teaspoonsful of a carrier oil.

homeopathy

Belladonna This may ease the initial stages of a rapidly developing sore throat with lots of inflammation and glandular swelling, if it is taken as soon as possible. The inside of the throat is likely to look bright red and there is a strong risk of developing a very high temperature.

Lachesis Sore throats and tonsillitis that specifically affect the left side, or move from left to right, are more likely to respond to this remedy. All symptoms feel worse when waking and, oddly, eating solid food appears to soothe a painful throat.

Hepar sulphuris calcareum (Hepar sulph.) Swollen glands associated with sore throats may need this remedy. Characteristic features of this remedy include a sharp pain as if something is sticking into the side of the throat. Exposure to cold draughts makes everything more sensitive and intense, while warmth in any form is soothing and pain-relieving.

nutritional approaches

In any situation where the body needs extra support to fight infection, it is a priority to increase your vitamin C intake by drinking fresh fruit juices and eating a lot of fresh fruit and vegetables

naturopathy

A generous fluid intake is essential in order to reduce feverishness and give the body maximum support by flushing out the by-products of infection.

western herbalism

For the localized relief of pain, try this soothing gargle.

Add 1 teaspoonful of sage to a cup of warm water. Leave to infuse for 60 seconds before straining and adding 1 teaspoonful of cider vinegar and honey.

colds

Although we generally regard the common cold as a minor health problem, a really heavy cold can make us feel wretched. The most common symptoms, which may occur in any combination, are listed below. Common triggers for catching a cold include lack of sleep and eating badly (both undermine immune system function), as well as being in close proximity to anyone who is sneezing and coughing.

common symptoms

- A sore, painful throat
- Sore, watery eyes
- Slight feverishness
- A streaming or scant nasal discharge or blocked nose
- Sneezing
- Pain and pressure in the cheekbones and/or above the eyes
- Ear pain
- A dry, irritating or loose, productive cough

conventional treatments

Most treatment is aimed at easing the discomfort of the major symptoms. Medications include painkillers, decongestants and/or formulas designed to loosen or suppress a persistent cough.

It helps to bear in mind that rest is one of our greatest allies in helping the body fight infection efficiently as well as staying in as stable a room temperature as possible. These simple measures ensure we're not diverting energy elsewhere that's needed to fight infection.

complementary treatments

Unlike conventional treatments, alternative and complementary therapies have much to offer in terms of supporting the body so that you can recover more quickly.

aromatherapy

To reduce fuzzy-headedness, add a drop or two of eucalyptus, tea tree or lavender essential oils to a tissue and inhale. Hold the tissue an inch or two from the nose, so that the concentrated oils do not come in contact with the delicate tissues of the nostrils.

homeopathy

Ferrum phosphoricum (Ferrum phos.) The earliest stage of a cold, where there is a sore throat that is very painful on swallowing and associated earache linked to muffled hearing, may respond to a few doses of Ferrum phos. When this remedy is indicated, the face may look alternately pale and flushed.

Aconite This is better for cold symptoms that come on quickly after exposure to dry, cold winds. The throat feels hot and dry, with marked thirst. The nasal passages feel correspondingly dry, with a general sense of restlessness and feverishness especially at night.

Belladonna Colds that come on violently and suddenly with a very high temperature with dry, hot skin will respond well. When this remedy is indicated, the skin, throat and ears are bright red and inflamed. As with Aconite, this remedy only helps during the early stages of a cold.

Natrum muriaticum (Natrum mur.) Head colds associated with the appearance of cold sores (suggesting that immune system function is at a low ebb) may be eased by this remedy. Characteristic symptoms include a nasal discharge that alternates between running like a tap or blocking the nostrils. Also, the lips and skin generally feel dry, taut and crack easily.

nutritional approaches

• Vitamin C has been shown to shorten the duration of a cold and discourage further problems from developing, such as swollen glands, sinus infection or residual catarrh. Take 500 mg of vitamin C twice daily for the duration of a cold. This can be taken in addition to the anti-oxidant supplement mentioned below.

• A combined supplement of vitamins A, C and E, plus the trace element selenium, is thought to support the immune system in fighting infection. Take it at the first sign of a sniffle.

naturopathy

• Avoid foods that are high in fat and difficult to digest. These can make you feel queasy and raise the body temperature even higher. Dairy products and sugar in particular make mucus congestion worse.

• Instead, keep up your water intake and opt for foods that are as light and easily digested as possible. Good choices include soups, steamed vegetables, fresh fruit and freshly squeezed fruit juices.

western herbalism

Echinacea has a well-deserved reputation for supporting the body in fighting viral infections. This appears to be linked to the balancing effect that this herbal medicine has on the immune system.

flu

Genuine flu is a very unpleasant, debilitating illness that will probably lay you up in bed for a couple of weeks. The symptoms, listed below, vary in intensity. It is worth taking enough time off in order to recover fully from a bout of the flu rather than rushing back on your feet too quickly. Otherwise you may risk a recurrence of the problem.

common symptoms

- Feverishness
- Shivers running up and down the spine
- Aching, heavy limbs
- Sore throat
- Headache
- Severe exhaustion
- Swollen glands
- Coughing spasms

conventional treatments

Treatments tend to focus on lowering a high temperature and providing pain relief in the form of paracetamol. Combination formulas may include other ingredients, such as decongestants. If a secondary infection of the throat or chest develops, antibiotics may be necessary.

complementary treatments

These can be immensely helpful in stimulating an efficient recovery and discouraging the development of complications. Choose any combination of the following.

aromatherapy

Vaporizing a few drops of eucalyptus, rosemary or peppermint essential oils in the sickroom helps to clear the air passages if mucus congestion is a problem, as well as creating a refreshing atmosphere.

homeopathy

Gelsemium Although by no means the only choice, this is the classic remedy for flu symptoms, such as shivers running up and down the spine, generalized aching in the muscles, heaviness of the legs and arms, and a headache that feels as if there is a tight band around the forehead.

Belladonna If the first stage of flu comes on very abruptly, with a very high temperature and flushed skin, this is the best remedy to consider. Confirmatory symptoms include restlessness, irritability, and sore ears and throat.

Mercurius Consider this once the fever has subsided, or if symptoms such as severe swelling in the glands, offensive-smelling sweat and thick green mucus develop.

Baptisia This is a good choice if the muscles ache a lot, with accompanying restlessness and exhaustion. There may be a marked sense of heaviness all over the body and difficulty in getting comfortable in bed. The throat is likely to be dark red, with a lot of swelling.

nutritional approaches

In the early stages of flu, it is more important to keep up your fluid intake than to eat, which is why it is natural to feel nauseous. Ideal fluids to opt for include still mineral water, herbal teas (either warm or chilled from the fridge) and freshly squeezed fruit juices.

naturopathy

• During the recovery phase, avoid putting extra strain on the liver which is one of the key detoxifying organs. Items to avoid at this stage include alcohol, coffee, high-fat foods and convenience foods containing artificial flavourings, colourings and preservatives.

• During the early stage of flu, you feel achy, shivery and altogether wiped out. Heed these signals and rest, since this is one of the most important things you can do to help your body fight infection.

western herbalism

• Sip a soothing herbal blend of tea to ease nausea and soothe your throat. Ideal herbs are peppermint or elderflower.

• Take Echinacea for the duration of the infection in order to support the immune system and thus recover as speedily as possible.

catarrh

When mucus secretions in the nose, throat and lungs are in balance, you should not really be aware of these areas. However, when you enter a phase of imbalance, where too much or too little mucus is being produced, any of the following symptoms can arise. Do bear in mind that if you are a smoker, giving up the habit is one of the most positive things you can do to discourage problems with catarrh.

common symptoms

- **Blocked, congested nasal passages**
- **Earache**
- **A constantly dripping nose**
- **A maddening, irritating need to constantly swallow or cough in order to clear the throat, especially before speaking**

conventional treatments

Minor problems with occasional catarrh that develop as a complication of a cold may be treated with decongestants.

complementary treatments

The following self-help measures will ease a one-off bout of catarrh associated with the tail-end of a cold.

aromatherapy

A couple of drops of eucalyptus, lavender or ravensara essential oils inhaled from a tissue will relieve nasal obstruction.

homeopathy

Natrum muriaticum (Natrum mur.) This is used for catarrh that is either watery and thin, or a bit jelly-like (like raw egg white). Catarrh is likely to flow freely after a bout of uncontrollable sneezing.

Kali bichromum (Kali bich.) This is indicated where symptoms include a stringy, greenish mucus that is extremely difficult to dislodge and an unpleasant smell in the nose from congealed mucus.

nutritional approaches

Support your body's first line of defence (the immune system) by including generous portions of the following in your diet: raw fruit, fresh vegetables, mixed salads, whole grains, garlic, onions, and filtered or still mineral water.

naturopathy

You should avoid dairy products and foods rich in sugar (see also Sinusitis, pages 130–131).

western herbalism

Gargle with a soothing, catarrh-busting infusion made from goldenrod, peppermint or elderflower, with a dash of lemon juice or honey added for flavour.

bad breath

As a one-off, bad breath may be no more than an embarrassment. However, persistent bad breath should not be ignored because it may indicate a more deep-seated health problem. If bad breath is beginning to be a regular feature of life, don't be tempted to rely on masking it by using strong-smelling sprays or mouthwashes. Instead, take this as a sign that a more deep-seated disorder needs to be dealt with.

common causes

- **Stomach upsets**
- **Dental problems, such as infected or unhealthy gums or tooth cavities**
- **Irritation of the stomach caused by too much strong coffee or alcohol**
- **Eating too many spicy foods**
- **Recurrent throat infections**

conventional treatments

A one-off bout of bad breath may respond to more scrupulous oral hygiene, using a mouthwash and/or mouth-freshening spray. If infection is an on-going problem, your doctor may advise tests to see whether you have a low-level throat infection. If you have any doubts about your teeth, a visit to the dentist may be productive.

complementary treatments

Once you have been checked over and possible causes have been eliminated, any of the following measures can help to freshen the breath.

homeopathy

Nux vomica This can restore the balance of the system by speeding up the detoxification process and is useful if bad breath is the result of a night of drinking, smoking and eating unwisely (especially if the food was highly spiced). Other symptoms include a classic morning-after headache and generally feeling short-fused, fragile and queasy.

naturopathy

This mouthwash can be useful for bad breath, especially if is related to a low-level throat infection. The resin used has strong, natural antibacterial properties.

Add 2 to 3 drops of benzoin to a cup of water.

sinusitis

The sinuses are cavities in the skull lying behind the eyes and cheekbones. Particularly after a bad cold, they can become inflamed and blocked with mucus, giving rise to this painful, distressing condition. Symptoms vary in intensity and generally include any combination of those listed below. Bear in mind that exposure to dry, cold winds can aggravate severe pain. So make a point of being well wrapped up on a chilly day.

common symptoms

- Pain that settles above and below the eyes and around the cheekbones
- A sense of discomfort and pressure in one or both of these areas when stooping or bending forwards
- Obstruction in one or both nostrils, with difficulty in shifting mucus when blowing the nose
- Recurrent headaches with a tired feeling behind the eyes
- A nasty taste in the mouth, often combined with an equally unpleasant smell in the nose
- Thin or thick yellowish green mucus

conventional treatments

Doctors usually prescribe a course of antibiotics in the first instance, sometimes combined with a decongestant. If you have recurring sinus infections that do not respond to this treatment, you may require minor surgery. This is a simple procedure that involves washing out the sinuses, thus encouraging them to drain more freely.

complementary treatments

Any of the following self-help measures can ease an acute episode of sinusitis. However, if this condition is firmly established or very severe, you should consult a trained practitioner.

aromatherapy

Make this naturally decongestant blend of essential oils and gently massage a little around the base of the nostrils and the throat.

Add 2 drops each of eucalyptus, pine and sweet marjoram to 2 teaspoonsful of carrier oil.

homeopathy

Hepar sulphuris calcareum (Hepar sulph.) Use this to ease sinus congestion that is more uncomfortable when there is the least draught of cold air. Mucus tends to be thick and yellowish green and, unusually, nasal obstruction feels worse rather than better when you are in the open air.

Kali bichromum (Kali bich.) This is better for sinus pain that is focused mainly on the bridge of the nose. It is indicated when symptoms include stringy, greenish mucus that is extremely difficult to dislodge and an unpleasant smell in the nose from congealed mucus.

Pulsatilla Sinus congestion and discomfort that sets in during the last stages of a cold, accompanied by a loose cough, may respond well to this remedy. Symptoms become more pronounced in a warm, stuffy room and tend to be most distressing at night. The mucus produced is characteristically thick and green.

naturopathy

• Get as much fresh air as possible, since this seems to soothe inflamed, blocked and congested nasal passages.

• Use a humidifier to counteract the dryness that results from living in a centrally heated environment. Alternatively, place a bowl of water by each radiator, topping them up as the water evaporates.

nutritional approaches

• Avoid dairy foods, which have a reputation for aggravating sinus congestion because of their tendency to stimulate mucus production. Treat sugary foods with caution for the same reason.

• Include as much fresh garlic in your diet as possible in order to benefit from its natural anti-viral and antibiotic properties. If an acute episode of sinusitis threatens, increase your intake by adding a garlic supplement in tablet or capsule form.

• Increase your intake of fresh, raw or lightly cooked fruit and vegetables during the cold and flu season. Bright red, yellow, orange and dark green fruits and vegetables are rich in anti-oxidants, as well as vitamins A, C and E, and have been shown to help our immune systems fight infection.

western herbalism

Take echinacea at the first twinge of sinus pain in order to help the body fight infection. Although very effective in supporting the immune system in fighting infection, Echinacea is thought to be most effective when taken for short courses at a time. It should not, therefore, be regarded as a long-term or permanent treatment.

ear pain

Earache is less common in adults than in children but sinusitis sometimes results in infection of the middle ear. Extremely painful and distressing, a severe ear infection may be accompanied by any of the symptoms listed below. If there is any sign of discharge from the affected ear, always seek a prompt medical opinion.

common symptoms

- **A muffled, full sensation in the ear**
- **Noises that can range from popping to cracking**
- **Sharp, stabbing or throbbing pains in the ear**
- **A general sense of malaise and feverishness**
- **Temporary loss of hearing and/ or balance**

conventional treatments

Treatment tends to focus on the use of painkillers and antibiotics in order to combat the infection. If general mucus congestion is aggravating a tendency to ear infections, a doctor may prescribe decongestants as well.

For severe cases of recurrent ear infection with mucus congestion in evidence, a minor surgical procedure may be suggested, which involves a tiny tube being inserted into the ear.

complementary treatments

Treatments can be especially helpful in discouraging the repeated emergence of ear infections but in order for them to work successfully, they should be given by a trained practitioner. The suggestions below are aimed at the short-term relief of ear pain and can be used safely alongside any conventional treatment.

cranial osteopathy

Recent research at the Oklahoma State University in the United States shows that osteopathic manipulation can reduce the incidence of ear infections in children aged 6 months to 6 years. Since this treatment appears to help children, adults may also benefit from a course of manipulation of this kind.

homeopathy

Chamomilla A few doses of this remedy can ease ear pain significantly. The pain is most likely to be combined with general feverishness and one cheek is often noticeably red, flushed and hot, while the other is contrastingly pale.

Belladonna Use this to soothe ear pain of rapid onset, with throbbing pain and inflammation and localized bright redness of the affected ear. The ear may be distinctly hot to the touch and the pain may be combined with a sore throat, swollen glands and a generally feverish state.

Aconite This is a specific remedy for ear pain that comes on suddenly after exposure to strong, dry, cold winds. The pain may be so severe that you feel on the verge of a panic attack.

nutritional approaches

• For any problems involving excessive mucus production and congestion, you should cut down on dairy products and sugary foods and drinks.

• Be aware that orange juice, because it is tart and acidic, may aggravate a painful throat and stimulate sensitive salivary glands. It may be best to avoid it if ear pain is accompanied by a sore throat and/or swollen glands in the face and neck.

naturopathy

• Hold a soothing warm compress gently against a painful ear. All you need is a hot-water bottle with a soft cover. Even simpler, wring out a face cloth after soaking it in hot water.

• Never poke an object into the ears, however blocked or itchy they may feel. It may provide some short-term relief but it can damage the ear in the long run. There is also a risk of the object going too far in to be retrieved.

western herbalism

A warm compress will be extra soothing and pain-relieving if it is soaked in an infusion of chamomile tea.

tinnitus

Tinnitus is a term used to describe a buzzing, hissing or ringing sensation in the ears that is not related to any obvious background noise. It can be very distressing and may be triggered by any of the features listed below. Unfortunately, the stress that is generated by the condition can be a significant factor in aggravating the symptoms. As a result, stress-management techniques should be a priority.

common triggers

- **A build-up of wax in the ears or removal of wax by syringing**
- **Hearing loss**
- **Stress-related conditions such as anxiety and/or depression**
- **High blood pressure**
- **Exposure to loud noise**
- **Use of certain drugs, such as aspirin, chloroquine or quinine**
- **Damage to the eustachian tube that runs from the nose to the ear**
- **Damage to the inner ear**
- **Alcohol**

conventional treatments

People often worry that their tinnitus may be due to a more serious condition, which is seldom the case. Unfortunately, anxiety and tension can aggravate the symptoms, so it is best to seek medical advice as soon as possible in order to put the mind at rest. If you have severe established tinnitis, a masker may help. This device fits into the ear, rather like a hearing aid, and provides low-level background sound or 'white noise' to distract you from the symptoms.

complementary treatments

This condition tends to be well established and chronic and, for effective treatment, you should consult an experienced alternative or complementary practitioner rather than trying to manage the situation yourself.

Suitable therapies from which to choose are listed below.

therapies to consider

Eastern therapies
- Chinese herbalism
- Shiatsu

Manipulative therapies
- Cranial osteopathy

Natural therapies
- Nutritional therapy
- Naturopathy
- Western herbalism
- Homeopathy

Active therapies
- Psychotherapy and counselling
- Relaxation techniques such as autogenic training
- Psychological and stress-management therapies

dizziness

As well as fluctuating blood sugar levels, low blood pressure and postural hypotension, there are two major ear conditions that cause dizziness (or vertigo as it is sometimes called), both associated with the inner ear. The first is Meniere's disease which is caused by an increase in the fluid balance and the second is labyrinthitis, which results from an infection.

common symptoms

Meniere's disease

- **Severe problems with balance**

- **Nausea and/or episodes of vomiting**

- **Hearing problems**

Labyrinthitis

- **Extreme dizziness**

- **Nausea and/or vomiting**

conventional treatments

Treatment of Meniere's disease involves drugs to reduce the amount of fluid in the inner ear and anti-nausea medication. Treatment for labyrinthitis is most likely to include bed rest and medication aimed at reducing nausea and vomiting.

complementary treatments

Realistically speaking, because both these conditions are so distressing, complementary treatments tend to be of most use after an acute attack, with a view to preventing further episodes. They can be of particular value if the condition is related to high stress levels. Periodic spells of severe dizziness can reduce confidence and heighten anxiety levels even in the most chilled-out individual. As a result, the objective assessment of an experienced practitioner of complementary medicine can be immensely reassuring.

therapies to consider

If you wish to consult a trained practitioner, consider one of the following:

Eastern therapies

- Acupressure

- Chinese herbalism

- Shiatsu

Manipulative therapies

- Reflexology

Natural therapies

- Aromatherapy

- Homeopathy

- Nutritional therapy

- Naturopathy

- Western herbalism

coughs

Coughs are usually a complication of a heavy cold or flu and can vary enormously in severity. Some coughs are no more than a tickle, while others seem to be raising phlegm from our boots! Remember, however, that the coughing reflex is a way of ridding the lungs of any congestion that would otherwise make it more difficult to breathe.

common symptoms

- Tickling, irritating sensation in the throat or upper chest
- A sense of tightness in the chest
- Regular spasms of coughing that may be productive (raising mucus) or dry and irritating
- Coughs may be accompanied by wheezing in the chest

conventional treatments

These usually take the form of cough medicines aimed at loosening or suppressing the cough, depending on whether it is dry and irritating, or productive. If the cough is part of a chest infection, antibiotics may be necessary.

complementary treatments

Many of these aim to support the coughing reflex so that we bring up mucus as easily, quickly and efficiently as possible.

aromatherapy

Make the following soothing aromatherapy blend to rub on the chest.

Add 4 drops of tea tree or eucalyptus essential oils to 2 tablespoonful of carrier oil.

homeopathy

Rumex This can help to soothe coughing spasms that are triggered by touching the throat, especially when coughing leads to choking spasms and breathlessness, and when breathing produces a raw, burning sensation in the chest.

Phosphorus Coughing spasms with tightness in the chest and yellow phlegm, and burning sensations in the chest with an alternating dry and loose cough that gets worse in the evenings may respond to this remedy.

Bryonia Dry, tickly coughs with a lot of irritation around the throat area and upper chest, and spasms that produce soreness will respond better to this remedy.

Pulsatilla Coughing spasms at the end of a heavy cold, alternating between dry and tickly and loose and productive, will do better with this remedy. Mucus from the throat and chest is likely to be thick and yellowish green.

nutritional approaches

• Increasing the amount of garlic in your diet can be of particular help for coughs. Garlic encourages the breakdown of mucus deposits and phlegm, and also has natural antibiotic properties. If you do not like the taste, try a supplement made from powdered garlic, preferably one that has a high allicin content.

• Avoid milky drinks before going to bed because dairy products in general (including cow's milk, cheese and cream) are thought to increase mucus production. This can make the chest much more congested, particularly when lying down.

naturopathy

• Go to sleep propped up by a few extra pillows so that mucus can drain more efficiently, and the chest can expand and relax more easily. Lying flat at night can lead to mucus build-up in the lungs.

• A steamy atmosphere, as in the shower, can give temporary relief to a dry, harsh cough, while a gentle walk in the fresh air can benefit loose, productive coughs. Use a humidifier at home and at work to combat an overly dry, centrally heated atmosphere, which can aggravate coughing spasms.

western herbalism

Try one of the natural cough medicines on the market that aim to loosen a dry or irritating cough.

bronchitis

Bronchitis develops when the mucus lining of the bronchial tubes in the lungs become irritated or inflamed. This may be a complication of a heavy cold or flu, or it may be a long-term problem that can seriously affect breathing patterns. It is also associated with smoking and air pollution. As a result, giving up smoking and avoiding regular contact with a smoky atmosphere should be a natural priority.

common symptoms

- **High fever**
- **Pain and tenderness in the upper area of the chest during a coughing bout**
- **Difficulty in taking a breath**
- **Constant coughing spasms that may produce grey, yellow or greenish phlegm**
- **Wheezing or rattling sounds in the chest**

conventional treatments

A one-off attack of bronchitis, with yellow phlegm, usually responds to rest and a course of antibiotics. If wheezing is marked, a bronchodilator (as used in asthma) may help to open up the airways.

complementary treatments

Any of the following self-help measures may be used alongside conventional medication in order to speed up recovery from an acute attack of bronchitis. If the problem is more established or recurring, it is worth consulting a trained complementary therapist in order to reduce any susceptibility to the problem.

naturopathy

• Rest during an attack is essential, ideally in surroundings that are neither too stuffy nor chilly. This helps the body to conserve its energy for fighting infection rather than using it to adjust to changing temperatures.

• Since an overly dry atmosphere can aggravate coughing bouts, use a humidifier or place a bowl of water near each radiator.

• Keep your body well hydrated by drinking plenty of filtered tap water or still mineral water, with a dash of added fresh fruit juice for the sake of variety. A high fluid intake supports the body's detoxifying mechanisms so that it can deal with infection more effectively.

• Avoid smoky places and if you are a smoker give up.

nutritional approaches

Whenever chest problems are an issue, you should avoid mucus-promoting dairy produce and sugary foods. Instead, opt for a primarily raw, fresh diet that includes plenty of fresh fruit and vegetables.

homeopathy

Rumex This soothes coughing spasms triggered by touching the throat and is indicated when coughing leads to choking spasms and breathlessness, and when breathing produces raw, burning feelings in the chest.

Phosphorus Coughing spasms with tightness in the chest and yellow phlegm may respond to this remedy. It may also be helpful where burning sensations in the chest alternate with a dry and loose cough that gets worse in the evenings.

Bryonia Dry, tickly coughs, with irritation around the throat area and upper chest and spasms producing soreness, will respond better to this remedy.

Pulsatilla Coughing spasms at the end of a heavy cold, alternating between dry, tickly and loose, productive, will do better with this remedy. Mucus from the throat and chest is likely to be thick and yellowish green.

asthma

This distressing condition often starts in childhood and clears up by the teenage years, but it sometimes remains a problem through adulthood. This health problem appears to be on the increase, affecting up to 1 in 7 people in the UK and Ireland. The figures for the US are somewhat lower, standing at 1 in 15. Symptoms vary enormously in severity and include any variation of the following.

common symptoms

- **Wheezing**
- **Coughing**
- **A sense of tightness in the chest, as if it is encased in a tight band**
- **Breathlessness that gets worse on contact with very cold air or when exercising**
- **Fast heartbeat**

conventional treatments

These concentrate on relaxing the air passages so that it becomes easier to breathe. Treatment of moderate asthma usually includes a steroid inhaler for use in the long term and a bronchodilator, which has a more immediate effect, for acute attacks.

Warning Never change the dosage of inhaled or oral steroids without consulting your doctor or you may suffer an adverse reaction.

complementary treatments

It should be stressed that the severe nature of an asthma attack means that self-treatment is out of the question. However, a trained practitioner of complementary medicine can provide effective treatment that will work alongside any conventional treatment. The following general advice can be helpful in cases of mild asthma.

practicalities

• Avoid smoky atmospheres and if you are a smoker give up.

• Learning a controlled breathing technique may help in the long term. Consider the Alexander technique, which focuses on correcting postural habits that may be counter-productive, or diaphragmatic breathing techniques that help you to make full use of your lung capacity.

• Swimming can be helpful provided the chlorine in the water does not make symptoms worse.

• Invest in anti-dust-mite covers for your bedding and replace curtains with blinds, and carpets with tiles.

therapies to consider

If you wish to consult a trained practitioner, consider one of the following:

• Chinese herbalism

• Homeopathy

• Nutritional therapy

• Western herbalism

hay fever

This irritating condition can ruin a good summer for hay-fever sufferers, who may feel as if they have a nasty cold that comes and goes throughout the season. The most common symptoms are listed below. Sufferers of allergic rhinitis are unfortunate in experiencing similar low-grade symptoms all year round. These symptoms are noticeably severe on waking and in the morning and usually include violent, repeated bouts of sneezing.

common symptoms

- Sore, watery eyes
- Itchy eyes with swelling of the eyelids after scratching or rubbing
- Light sensitivity
- Sneezing (often violent and repeated)
- Soreness or itching of the throat
- Itchy ears or the roof of the mouth
- Wheezing and/or tightness in the chest

conventional treatments

Antihistamines may reduce the worst of the symptoms. If you have asthma that gets worse during the hay-fever season, your doctor may review your inhaler to give extra coverage. He or she may also offer practical advice on avoiding exposure to your allergies whenever possible, such as turning on the air filters when driving or wearing close-fitting sunglasses on windy, sunny days.

complementary treatments

Although they can provide acute support during the hay-fever season, most practitioners will want to see a hay-fever patient during the autumn and winter so that they can devise a preventive treatment to help the immune system work in a more balanced way. During the hay-fever season, any of the following self-help measures may provide additional support.

practicalities

If you have been tested for allergies and know that you are sensitive to house-dust mites and their droppings, vacuum your house daily. It may also be helpful to put mite-proof covers on your bedding.

homeopathy

Apis This can be immensely helpful in reducing any puffiness and swelling around the eyes. The affected area is likely to look rosy pink and waterlogged, but will usually feel temporarily better after bathing.

Euphrasia If your eyes water profusely and the tears burn and smart, it is time to consider this remedy. Your nose may run in sympathy but the discharge, in contrast to that from the eyes, is not so uncomfortable.

Allium cepa This is more suitable for a streaming, clear nasal discharge that makes the upper lip and base of the nostrils feel sore and tender, and where the eyes water profusely, but the tears are not too uncomfortable.

Sabadilla Hay-fever symptoms that arise from the smell or even the thought of flowers may be eased by this remedy. Episodes of sneezing are accompanied by a dry, tickling sensation in the nose that seems to spread across the body.

nutritional approaches

Studies suggest that a deficiency of B-complex vitamins may increase our vulnerability to allergic reactions. Consider taking a precautionary supplement of B-complex vitamins before and during the hay-fever season.

naturopathy

• Bathe the eyes and face in cool water to give temporary relief.

• Sensible practical steps include wearing sunglasses to protect sensitive eyes in strong sunlight and staying indoors when pollen or pollution counts are exceptionally high.

• Avoid exposure to any irritants that may trigger symptoms (this includes gardening). Common triggers include dust, animal fur, perfumes and fungal spores from mould and damp.

western herbalism

• Sensitive, sore, itchy eyes can be soothed by bathing them in this diluted Euphrasia tincture. The simplest way of doing this is to soak a couple of clean cottonwool pads in the solution, and gently place them over your closed eyes while you put your feet up.

Add 4 drops of Euphrasia tincture to 150 ml (5 fl oz) of cooled, boiled water.

If you don't have any Euphrasia tincture to hand, use cool cucumber slices instead, or boiled, cooled Indian teabags. Both can have a very soothing effect in the short term.

constipation

There is nothing like a bout of constipation to make us feel sluggish! It may not be the most glamorous thing to think about, but the regularity and efficiency of our bowel movements are important, if we want to enjoy a state of optimum health and glowing vitality. This is because the effective detoxification of our bodies depends on healthy bowel function. Symptoms of constipation include any combinations of the following.

common symptoms

- **Infrequent, incomplete stools that involve straining or are painful to pass**
- **Abdominal bloating and discomfort**
- **Headaches**
- **Tiredness and lethargy**
- **Loss of appetite**

conventional treatments

This usually involves dietary advice and the use of laxatives. However, while laxatives can be used occasionally, they should not be adopted as a long-term strategy because they can make the bowel less efficient. This can lead to malabsorption, especially if it results in frequent diarrhoea.

complementary treatments

Any combination of the following measures can be used to deal with occasional bouts of mild constipation. However, you should consult a trained practitioner if your digestive system as a whole is sluggish (triggering problems of indigestion and irregular bowel movements).

aromatherapy

A blend of fennel, marjoram or rosemary essential oils, diluted in a carrier oil, can feel very soothing when massaged over the abdomen. Since constipation can be made more of a problem by feeling tense or stressed, this measure should have a soothing, relaxing effect.

homeopathy

Bryonia This may ease constipation associated with a state of low-level dehydration. Associated symptoms include headache, dry mouth and a general sense of inactivity in the bowel, with no desire to 'go' at all.

Nux vomica General toxicity and sluggishness in the digestive tract caused by too much alcohol, too many cigarettes, an unwise mixture of food, too much partying and too little sleep may respond better to this remedy. There may also be a maddening desperation to 'go' but with very little being achieved. This remedy is also excellent for easing constipation that is worsened by stress.

nutritional approaches

• To keep the digestive tract functioning smoothly, it is essential to include enough complex, unrefined carbohydrates in the daily diet. Ensure a healthy supply by opting for brown rice (and rice cakes made from organic brown rice), wholemeal products, fresh fruit, raw vegetables, dried fruit and freshly squeezed vegetable and fruit juices.

• Avoid the following whenever possible because they have a reputation for slowing down efficient elimination from the bowel: convenience foods, any products made from refined white flour, white rice, cheese and red meat.

naturopathy

• A regular daily intake of dietary fibre will guard against constipation. Eat high-fibre foods such as fresh fruit (especially apples, pears, plums and fresh figs), fresh vegetables and wholegrain products, such as wholmeal bread and brown rice cakes.

• An estimated 70 per cent of cases of constipation appear to be linked to insufficient fluid intake. Therefore, you should drink a minimum of five large glasses of filtered or still mineral water each day to ensure the easy passage of bowel contents.

• Remember that pain-killers involving combinations of paracetamol and codeine can contribute to stubborn constipation.

western herbalism

To ease a one-off bout of constipation, drink one cupful of the following preparation three times a day after meals.

Add 2 teaspoonsful of psyllium seeds to a cup of warm water and stir well. Leave to stand for 5 minutes before stirring well again. Flavour with lemon and honey.

hiatus hernia

This condition involves the acid contents of the stomach washing back into the gullet because of a weakness in the diaphragm. Someone with hiatus hernia may also have heartburn (or indigestion) but the odd bout of heartburn (or indigestion) it doesn't automatically imply hiatus hernia. It is especially common in women who are overweight or suffering from a temporary weight gain, as, for example, during pregnancy.

common symptoms

- Discomfort and/or burning in the chest, triggered or made more intense by bending over
- Frequent bouts of acidity, during which a small amount of acid rises into the throat (especially when stooping)
- Belching and burping

conventional treatments

Treatment focuses on drugs that either temporarily increase the surface tension of the stomach contents or speed the stomach contents on its way, so that stomach acid is less likely to wash back into the gullet.

complementary treatments

The following self-help measures will help ease the symptoms of hiatus hernia in the short term. For more long-term relief, you should consult a trained practitioner.

nutritional approaches

Apart from avoiding items that irritate the stomach lining and increase acid production (such as coffee, alcohol, tea and cigarettes), it is worth losing a few pounds if being overweight is contributing to the problem.

western herbalism

A warm drink of slippery elm powder mixed with milk can ease any digestive discomfort. You can take slippery elm in tablet form if you are unable to eat dairy products.

naturopathy

- If you have no history of swollen ankles, it may help to prop up the head of your bed slightly or to sleep propped up on two or three square continental pillows.

- Avoid bending and stooping immediately after a meal, when the stomach is full, which will prevent acid washing back into your gullet.

gallstones

Once we reach our 50s, many of us may be unwittingly harbouring a few gallstones. It is only when they begin to move that we become aware of them. If this happens, the gall bladder may become inflamed and swollen, leading to the following symptoms. Often gallstones can be symptomless, with many of us only being told we have them as a result of a scan carried out for other reasons.

common symptoms

- **Severe pain on the right side beneath the rib cage, between the shoulderblades or in the right shoulder**
- **Nausea and vomiting**
- **A yellowish tinge to the whites of the eyes, skin and/or urine**

conventional treatments

Initially, doctors tend to offer dietary advice as a way of managing the condition. However, if attacks of pain and vomiting start to occur on a frequent basis, they may suggest surgical removal of the gall bladder or shattering of the gall stones with ultra sound.

complementary treatments

This situation does not lend itself to self-treatment, largely because of the severe pain involved in an acute episode of gallstone colic. It is therefore best to consult a trained alternative or complementary practitioner. Nevertheless, the following lifestyle hints may be helpful as a background strategy.

nutritional approaches

- Avoid foods associated with gallstone colic, such as full fat cheese, cream, red meat, chocolate and deep-fried foods.

- Instead, opt for gall-bladder friendly foods, such as plenty of fresh fruit, vegetables, whole grains, pulses and small amounts or poultry and fish. Note that certain foods appear to help regulate the concentration of bile salts in the body which can leave us vulnerable to gall stones. These include artichokes, asparagus, kelp and barley water.

therapies to consider

If you wish to consult a trained practitioner, consider one of the following:

- Naturopathy
- Chinese herbalism
- Nutritional therapy
- Western herbalism
- Homeopathy

indigestion and heartburn

Since the symptoms of these two conditions often overlap, it makes sense to consider them together. They include the following. Bear in mind that should you experience recurrent bouts of indigestion for no obvious reason, this is something that should be investigated by your doctor.

common symptoms

- **A heavy, uncomfortable feeling in the stomach**
- **Burning sensations behind the breastbone**
- **Acid reflux with a burning liquid washing up into the throat (see also hiatus hernia, page 146)**
- **Hiccups**
- **Nausea**
- **Belching and flatulence with 'repeating' of recently eaten food**

conventional treatments

Drug treatment may involve antacids aimed at diluting the production of excess stomach acid or a group of drugs called H2 blockers, which also work on acid secretion in the stomach.

A test may also be carried out to check for the presence of Pylori. This is a bacterium that can leave us more vulnerable to the production of a stomach ulcer. Should this be found to be the case, antibiotic treatment will be given.

complementary treatments

Any of the following self-help measures can be used to deal with a mild episode of indigestion or heartburn. For more established or severe patterns of stomach disorder, you should consult a trained practitioner who will aim to rebalance digestive function at a more profound level.

aromatherapy

Make this soothing massage blend which you can apply gently to your belly and abdomen in slow, circular movements.

Add 2 drops of peppermint, ginger, mandarin and Roman chamomile essential oils to 2 teaspoonsful of carrier oil.

homeopathy

Pulsatilla This may ease indigestion and queasiness caused by eating too many rich, fatty foods. This remedy is indicated by a characteristic burping and 'repeating' of food eaten a couple of hours earlier.

Bryonia This remedy is better for general uneasiness, with a sense of weight in the stomach and nausea that develops soon after eating. Characteristic symptoms include heartburn and acidity with a marked thirst for cold drinks.

Arsenicum album Burning pains with marked queasiness and possibly diarrhoea, which are soothed by sipping warm drinks, may respond well to this remedy. It can be especially effective in relieving any distress that these symptoms cause at night.

Lycopodium Stress-related digestive uneasiness, characterized by acid reflux and stubborn heartburn, with abdominal bloating and rumbling, gurgling sounds, may respond to this remedy. It is also indicated where there is loss of appetite after eating even a small quantity of food.

In such a situation the entire digestive tract may be out of balance, with a tendency to alternating episodes of constipation and diarrhoea.

nutritional approaches

Avoid foods and drinks with a reputation for aggravating stomach discomfort, such as items made from refined white sugar and flour (thought to increase acidity) and stomach irritants such as alcohol, strong tea and coffee, and cigarettes.

naturopathy

• Consider your eating patterns as well as the quality of what you eat. Try to eat in a relaxed way, avoiding eating on the run or while working at a computer.

• Eat small amounts of nutritious food at regular intervals and include a bowl of bio-yogurt each day to maintain the balance of the intestinal flora of the gut.

western herbalism

• Sipping a cup of ginger tea or nibbling on a piece of crystallized ginger can do a surprising amount to ease nausea and indigestion.

Warning Ginger is best avoided by people with stomach ulcers.

• For flatulence, try this soothing, herbal infusion.

Add 1 teaspoonful of fennel, peppermint or lemon balm to a cup of hot water, leave to stand for 15 minutes and straining before drinking.

haemorrhoids

Haemorrhoids, or piles as they are more commonly known, are dilated varicose veins in the rectum. They are seldom serious unless they prolapse (drop out of the rectum) but can still be painful and distressing. They often result from chronic constipation, especially during pregnancy. Alternatively, they may result from a difficult labour. Symptoms, which are hard to miss, are listed below.

common symptoms

- **Bright red bleeding from the rectum after passing a stool (often after straining)**
- **Itching, soreness or irritation of the rectum**
- **Prolapsed haemorrhoids may be extra-sensitive**

conventional treatments

Medications include topical applications, such as creams to soothe painful, itchy haemorrhoids. If the haemorrhoids are especially severe and interfering with quality of life, surgical removal may be necessary.

complementary treatments

Any of the following self-help measures may help to ease the pain and distress of a mild but acute episode of haemorrhoid pain.

aromatherapy

Adding a few drops of myrrh, cypress or frankincense essential oils to a warm bath may be very soothing.

homeopathy

Hamamelis This will soothe the prickling, stinging pains of haemorrhoids that tend to bleed very easily.

Alumina If pronounced itching occurs after a bowel movement, or passing even the softest of stools involves an unusual amount of straining, consider this remedy.

nutritional approaches

Make sure that constipation does not aggravate the condition (see Constipation, pages 144–45) and include the following items in your diet in order to give things a kick start: prunes, dried apricots, and/or brown rice cakes.

naturopathy

Applying cool compresses or bathing in warm water may substantially relieve the pain and itching in the short term. Apply warm and cool compresses alternately to the affected area or add a handful of sea salt to a warm bath.

western herbalism

Some herbal creams provide an excellent alternative to the chemically based creams associated with conventional medicines. These creams contain natural ingredients, such as horse chestnut, witch hazel or aloe in a soothing base.

irritable bowel syndrome

This catch-all term covers an astonishingly wide variety of digestive symptoms, which can include any combination of the following in varying degrees of severity. Stress is regarded as one of the main triggers of IBS, after aggravating symptoms. Additional triggers may include food sensitivities (especially to wheat and dairy foods) and a diet that is unbalanced with regard to fibre intake.

symptoms

- **Nausea**
- **Heartburn**
- **Indigestion**
- **Flatulence and belching**
- **Irregular bowel movements, possibly alternating between diarrhoea and constipation**
- **Cramping, colicky pains**
- **Bloating and distention of the abdomen**

conventional treatments

Treatment may involve any of a variety of drugs, as well as those mentioned for indigestion and heartburn (see pages 148–149). They include anti-spasmodic drugs to encourage smooth bowel movement, bulking agents used to soften stools and drugs aimed at controlling diarrhoea.

complementary treatments

For long-term problems of irritable bowel syndrome, you should consult a trained practitioner. They should be in a position to advise you about lifestyle changes that may help to counteract the symptoms. In addition, they have at their disposal a range of medicines that may gently encourage the digestive tract to work more smoothly. In the short-term, the following self-help measures may prove useful.

nutritional approaches

Although stress is considered to play a major role in triggering or aggravating irritable bowel syndrome, diet may also be important. Foods that are thought to aggravate the condition include wheat, dairy foods and items rich in unrefined white sugar. If you suspect this may be happening, try an elimination diet for three weeks, cutting out any possibly offending item. If your digestion improves noticeably, re-introduce the food and note how you react. If symptoms get worse or re-appear, avoid that food again. If the same pattern emerges for a second time, you may well be sensitive to this food.

homeopathy

Nux vomica Irritable bowel symptoms brought on by stress and junk foods may respond well to this remedy. It is helpful where bowel spasms are accompanied by pain that is more intense when any sudden jarring movement occurs.

Argenticum nitricum (Argent. nit) If sugary foods obviously make the symptoms more noticeable or severe, this remedy is worth considering, especially if there is a tendency to diarrhoea, with lots of noisy wind that travels in an upward and downward direction.

Lycopodium This remedy is helpful when irritable bowel syndrome is noticeably linked to stress and anxiety about an important forthcoming event, where there is a marked tendency for alternate bouts of constipation and diarrhoea, and a corresponding bloating in the abdomen.

Colocynthis Consider this remedy if the discomfort and cramping pains of irritable bowel syndrome are temporarily eased by bending double. This remedy is strongly indicated when watery diarrhoea tends to be triggered by anger or bouts of emotional stress, and when waves of abdominal cramps follow eating and/ or drinking.

western herbalism

• Aloe vera juice has a positive reputation for soothing and regularizing the digestive tract. If you find it unappetizing, try it in capsule form.

• A warm infusion of peppermint or chamomile tea may also calm down an upset bowel, especially if a little ginger is added.

yoga

Since irritable bowel syndrome is often regarded as a stress-related problem, it is worth considering taking up a stress-reducing system of movement, such as yoga. This helps not only to condition a neglected body, but also to calm and relax the mind by the use of controlled breathing techniques.

food-poisoning

Anyone who has experienced a bad dose of food-poisoning will remember how exhausted and awful they felt while the bug was making its way out of their system. Symptoms vary in duration and severity, and may include any variation of the following. Should vomiting and diarrhoea occur together in the very young or the elderly, do watch out for signs of dehydration which demand immediate medical attention.

symptoms

- **Vomiting**
- **Nausea**
- **Diarrhoea**
- **Stomach and/or abdominal cramps**
- **Exhaustion**
- **Perspiration which can leave you feeling hot or clammy**

conventional treatments

Treatments tend to focus on putting fluids back into the body, rather than suppressing the vomiting or diarrhoea. This is significant because, however unpleasant the vomiting and diarrhoea may be (especially if they occur together), they are the means by which the body rids itself of infection. As a result, suppression of the symptoms means that the infection will go on for longer.

complementary treatments

Self-help measures for a simple case of food-poisoning can be one of the most impressive experiences for the newcomer to complementary therapies. When well-chosen, they can speed up recovery and make you feel generally much better within an incredibly short space of time.

nutritional approaches

Once the vomiting and diarrhoea have subsided, it is important to take easily digestible foods and drinks. Opt for lots of water, soups, lightly steamed vegetables, freshly squeezed fruit juices (not citrus) and natural yoghurt. Avoid citrus fruit (too acidic), tea and coffee (stomach irritants), and fatty or spicy foods, which will either be too irritating or difficult to digest (and therefore more likely to trigger fresh bouts of queasiness).

naturopathy

The first priority in treating food-poisoning is to ensure that you do not become dehydrated. To guard against this, you should take frequent small sips of water rather than attempting to drink larger quantities at one time. In this way, the stomach is less likely to vomit it up again quickly, because larger amounts of fluid increase stomach pressure, making vomiting more likely.

western herbalism

• Spices such as ginger are not only useful condiments but can also soothe an upset, queasy stomach. Make a soothing infusion by adding a small amount of freshly grated ginger root to a teapotful of hot water. Leave to stand for 15 minutes before straining off the soothing liquid.

• Sipping an infusion of chamomile, fennel or peppermint can help to settle a disordered stomach after a bout of food-poisoning. Slippery elm can also be immensely helpful in calming a sensitive stomach after a bout of food-poisoning.

aromatherapy

Gently rubbing the abdomen with a massage blend of chamomile or geranium essential oils may be soothing.

homeopathy

Arsenicum album This is a useful remedy when diarrhoea and vomiting occur together. It also helps to relieve the symptoms of chilliness, restlessness and anxiety that accompany episodes of vomiting.

Veratrum album This is another remedy that soothes simultaneous diarrhoea and vomiting. The main way of distinguishing between this remedy and Arsenicum relates to thirst levels. Veratrum is indicated when there is an unquenchable thirst for ice-cold water, which unfortunately tends to be vomited up very soon after drinking.

Ipecacuanha (Ipecac.) This may ease the dreadful nausea that is not relieved slightly or temporarily by vomiting, and which feels much worse for even the slightest movement. In addition, the abdomen may feel bloated and uncomfortable, with colicky, intermittent pains.

cystitis

Caused by an infection or inflammation of the bladder, cystitis occurs more frequently in women than men. Apart from being painful, the constant need to pass urine can be both inconvenient and embarrassing, especially if cystitis occurs on a regular basis. If symptoms do not respond to complementary self-help measures within 24–28 hours, or if the pain becomes more severe, seek professional medical opinion.

common symptoms

- **A general sense of feverishness and malaise**
- **Pain at the beginning, during or at the end of passing urine**
- **A troublesome, bearing-down sensation located in the lower abdomen and/or lower back**
- **Strong, dark, concentrated urine**
- **A constant urge to pass urine or slight, involuntary dribbling of urine**

conventional treatments

Over-the-counter preparations focus on making it less painful to pass urine. If bouts of cystitis are more severe or established, a doctor may arrange for a urine test to determine the nature of the infection before prescribing a course of antibiotics.

complementary treatments

Any of the following self-help measures can relieve a mild to moderate bout of cystitis, especially if used at the first twinge of pain. However, if you have a tendency to severe cystitis, you should consult an experienced practitioner.

practicalities

• Never put off the urge to pass water and take time to empty the bladder completely, rather than finishing too swiftly. Both these common habits can make us more vulnerable to bladder infections.

• After emptying the bowels, take care to wipe from front to back, rather back to front, in order to reduce the chances of cross-infection.

aromatherapy

A massage with the following blend of essential oils can significantly soothe the discomfort and distress of acute cystitis. If you have difficulty obtaining these oils, consult a practitioner who will be able to make up a blend for you.

Add 2 drops of tea tree, lavender, niaouli and thymus linanol to 4 teaspoonsfuls of carrier oil.

homeopathy

Cantharis This is one the most frequently indicated remedies for the classic symptoms of cystitis, such as burning and stinging before, during and after passing water, and a constant urge to empty the bladder, although you only pass a small amount of urine each time.

Sarsaparilla This is a specific for cystitis with scalding, burning pains that are noticeably worse at the end of urinating; starting the flow may be relatively pain-free.

Staphysagria Use this remedy to soothe the discomfort and distress of cystitis that develops after love-making or being catheterized for surgery. When symptoms are at their height, it may seem impossible to fully empty the bladder because of the pain.

naturopathy

• Make it a priority to avoid constipation, which can aggravate the general discomfort of cystitis. Do this by drinking at least five large glasses of filtered water a day (which will also make passing urine less painful) and increase the proportion of fibre-rich items in your diet. Avoid strawberries, citrus fruit, spinach, grapes, tomatoes and raw carrots, which can aggravate the symptoms of cystitis.

• Drinking home-made barley water makes the urine less acidic and therefore less painful to pass.

Add 2 tablespoonsful of pearl barley to a pan containing 1 litre (about 2 pints) of cold water. Bring it to the boil and strain off the liquid, which should be cooled in the fridge.

western herbalism

• Sipping a cup of warm chamomile tea may soothe some of the cramping muscle spasms of cystitis.

• Drinking a small glass of cranberry juice every couple of hours also seems to make the urine less acidic and less painful to pass. Once an acute episode is over, continuing to drink a glass a day may stop the urine becoming too acidic again.

kidney infections

In most cases, kidney infections are the result of an infection that has been spread from the bladder. Because of their severity, symptoms tend to be fairly obvious. Do make a point of dealing promptly with bladder infections with this in mind, especially if you have a previous history of kidney infections.

common symptoms

- **Pain that moves from the sides and back to the groin**
- **Frequent painful urination**
- **High fever**
- **Severe shivering**
- **Vomiting**
- **Marked chilliness**
- **Concentrated, pink and/or cloudy urine**

conventional treatments

If a urine test confirms an infection, you will need a course of antibiotics. If this does not completely clear up the symptoms, you may need another urine test to check for residual infection.

complementary treatments

Because of the severity of the symptoms, conventional treatment will probably be your first resort but you may then choose to consult an experienced complementary therapist, especially if you have a recurring tendency to kidney infections. There are a number of practical measures that you can take during the course of this treatment.

practicalities

- Increase your fluid intake to about 2 litres (3½ pints) of water a day.

- Cut down on protein and salt in the diet, since both put extra strain on the kidneys.

- Avoid foods that are difficult to digest until the acute attack is over; heavy, fatty foods put more strain on the digestive organs, increasing nausea and making it more likely that your temperature will go up.

therapies to consider

If you wish to consult a trained practitioner, consider one of the following:

Eastern therapies
- Chinese herbalism

Natural therapies
- Naturopathy
- Nutritional therapy
- Homeopathy
- Western herbalism

kidney stones

These deposits in the kidney tubules consist of salts which have been filtered from the fluid that passes through the kidneys. The larger ones, because they stay in one place, do not give rise to any symptoms. However, the smaller ones can travel through the kidney, producing severe and unpleasant symptoms. Some conditions can trigger the production of kidney stones.

common symptoms

- **Agonizing pain that travels from the sides to the groin**
- **Trembling and sweating**
- **Vomiting**
- **Restlessness**

common triggers

- **Repeated kidney infections**
- **Gout**
- **Too little fluid intake over the long term**

conventional treatments

If kidney stones are a recurring problem, your doctor may arrange for a scan or X-ray of the kidneys in order to establish whether there are any more waiting to move. If this is the case, you may need ultra-sound treatment to shatter the stones or surgery to remove them.

complementary treatments

Once the kidney stones have been passed, you may wish to consider complementary treatment to prevent the problem recurring.

practicalities

It is essential to drink enough water (approximately 2–3 litres, or 4–6 pints, a day) when the production of kidney stones is an issue. This can help flush out the kidneys on a regular basis.

therapies to consider

If you wish to consult a trained practitioner, consider one of the following:

Eastern therapies
- Ayurveda
- Chinese herbalism

Natural therapies
- Homeopathy
- Nutritional therapy
- Western herbalism

nutritional therapy

It may help to cut down on foods that are high in white sugar and salt, both of which are associated with the production of kidney stones. Also avoid foods that are high in oxalates. These foods include beetroot, rhubarb, chocolate and strawberries. On the positive side, cranberries and asparagus may help the body to break up oxalic acid crystals.

stress incontinence

This is most likely to occur as a result of pregnancy (especially if closely spaced) or multiple births. Signs of stress incontinence may also become noticeable from middle age onwards, as the ligaments that support the womb become less toned. Temporary stress incontinence may occur during a serious chest infection or bronchitis, because of the severity of the coughing bouts.

common symptoms

- Involuntary dribbling of urine when coughing, sneezing, laughing or exercising
- Backache, constipation and difficulty in passing urine (if stress incontinence is associated with a prolapsed bladder)
- An irritating urge to urinate, even when the bladder is virtually empty

conventional treatments

For mild bouts of stress incontinence that are related to certain activities, such as exercising, the use of incontinence pads may be sufficient. Pelvic-floor exercises may also improve the situation (see opposite). It may be wise to ask your doctor for a urine test in order to rule out the presence of a low-level urinary tract infection.

complementary treatments

Any of the following measures may help a mild tendency to stress incontinence. Do bear in mind that stress incontinence symptoms don't have to be an on-going, chronic problem, but can occur as a short-lived symptoms associated with a severe cough.

practicalities

• Daily pelvic-floor exercises (Kegel exercises) may noticeably improve mild or infrequent stress incontinence, and you can do them anywhere and at any time. Focus on the muscles that come into play when you try to stop passing water, then consciously contract and relax them repeatedly.

• Pilates and yoga can be useful in promoting a general sense of improved muscle tone and body awareness.

homeopathy

Gelsemium A sense of heaviness in the bladder and a constant urge to pass water can be helped by this remedy. Symptoms may be aggravated by tension, stress or anxiety.

Causticum This can relieve stress incontinence associated with very severe coughing or sneezing bouts and general muscle weakness.

Pulsatilla Where symptoms of mild stress incontinence follow pregnancy and childbirth, you should consider this remedy. Discomfort in the bladder is noticeably more severe when resting or lying down at night.

Sepia This remedy is strongly indicated where stress incontinence is combined with a marked bearing-down sensation in the abdomen and a sense of mental, emotional and physical exhaustion.

naturopathy

In hydrotherapy, alternating hot and cold Sitz baths are reputed to improve muscle tone and overall circulation to the pelvic area. You can do this simply at home. All you need are two large bowls, one of hot water and one of cold. First make sure that your bathroom is comfortably warm so that you do not get chilled. Cover the top half of your body in a warm towel and sit in the hot water, ensuring that it covers the pelvic area completely, while putting your feet in the cold water. Stay in this position for 3 minutes, then swap over. Do this two or three times, always ending up with your feet in cold water.
Warning Do not use this technique if you have a heart or circulatory problems. If in doubt, always ask your family doctor.

western herbalism

An infusion of horsetail will strengthen and improve the tone of the bladder. Add half a teaspoonful to a cup of hot water and take twice daily.
Warning Avoid long-term use and during pregnancy.

pre-menstrual syndrome

Pre-menstrual syndrome (PMS) can adversely affect a woman's mental, emotional and physical well-being. It commonly affects 40 per cent of women, while breast changes during the menstrual cycle affect up to 70 per cent. Symptoms vary in range and intensity – some women are only mildly affected on an infrequent basis while others experience a dramatic change from mid-cycle (ovulation) onwards.

common symptoms

- **Fatigue**
- **Mood swings**
- **Lack of concentration**
- **Poor coordination**
- **Breast tenderness and enlargement**
- **Oily skin that is prone to spots**
- **Fluid retention**
- **Food cravings (especially for salt and sugar)**
- **Recurrent headaches**
- **Thrush**
- **Poor sleep pattern**
- **Pain at ovulation**
- **Cramping pains before or at the onset of a period**
- **Lowered libido**

conventional treatments

These usually aim to lower the severity of the pain or reduce blood loss. If a blood test shows any severe hormone imbalance, you may need drugs to restore the balance. Progesterone treatment (supplements of a female sex hormone) is another controversial option. A localized problem such as severe fluid retention may require diuretic medication.

complementary treatments

All the measures described below can be helpful in gently easing the symptoms of PMS. They can be used alongside any of the conventional treatments outlined above.

practicalities

Research in the United States shows that a walk in the sunshine can boost the production of serotonin (a brain chemical that makes us feel good). Often a daily 20-minute stroll is all that is needed to lift a 'blue' mood.

aromatherapy

To soothe erratic mood swings that build up as the onset of a period gets closer, use the following massage blend. Alternatively, vaporize the oils in a burner to create a fragrant, calming atmosphere.

Add 3 drops of fennel and geranium to 4 drops of grapefruit essential oil and 1 tablespoonful of carrier oil, such as sweet almond, avocado, jojoba or wheatgerm oil.

homeopathy

When choosing a homeopathic remedy, remember that it needs to match your symptoms as closely as possible in order to obtain the best results.

Lachesis This is helpful for severe symptoms of PMS that start at ovulation, build progressively in intensity as the onset of a period gets closer and magically lift as soon as the flow starts. Common symptoms relieved by this remedy are left-sided migraines and headaches, and insomnia.

Sepia When the 'blues' descend or when you lack energy and your libido is markedly low, consider this remedy.

Pulsatilla This is helpful if you feel sad, weepy and emotionally vulnerable. It is also useful for irregular periods and pre-menstrual headaches and thrush.

nutritional approaches

• To balance mood swings, eat little and often (to balance blood sugar levels) and opt for foods that do not produce a sugar rush. Try unsweetened, natural bio-yoghurt, apples, pears, rye bread and brown rice.

• Avoid items that aggravate the symptoms, such as coffee, tea, alcohol, fizzy drinks, heavily salted snacks and fatty foods containing large amounts of hydrogenated oils.

• Remember that the phytoestrogens in soya products help prevent breast tenderness, while essential fatty acids (in oily fish such as salmon and mackerel, and in flaxseed oil) have a positive effect on hormone balance.

western herbalism

• According to research published in the *British Medical Journal* in 2001, a daily supplement of *Agnus castus* can ease breast discomfort, abdominal bloating and mood swings. This has a positive action on the pituitary gland, helping to balance the production of sex hormones.

• Ease fluid retention by drinking dandelion tea, which may also reduce symptoms of breast tenderness and abdominal bloating.

• Sip lemon verbena tea to banish headaches and tension.

• Drink a cup of peppermint or fennel tea to relieve digestive problems associated with PMS.

painful periods

Women may be more prone to painful or difficult periods at particular times, such as at the onset of menstruation or when they are approaching the menopause, when periods may change their nature quite noticeably. Other problems associated with a tendency to painful periods are listed below. Puberty can also be a time when periods are painful and irregular until a regular cycle has had time to establish itself.

common problems

- **Diarrhoea**
- **Clamminess**
- **Dizziness and disorientation**
- **Severe headaches**
- **Mood swings, such as tearfulness or irritability**
- **Fainting**
- **Nausea and vomiting**
- **A sense of being physically drained**

conventional treatments

These usually include pain-killing medication, to be taken as soon as the pain starts. This works by relaxing the muscles or inhibiting the contractions of the womb. The contraceptive pill may also be prescribed.

complementary treatments

Any of the following measures can be used alongside conventional treatments.

practicalities

For drug-free treatment of pain, try a TENS machine. Simple to use, it consists of a battery-operated unit, smaller than a personal stereo, and two to four adhesive pads, which are attached by wires. Apply the pads to the area where the pain is centred. Switch on the machine and you will feel a temporary, mild, tingling sensation that should swiftly disappear, along with the pain. TENS machines appear to work by producing a low-level electrical stimulation that blocks or slow downs the passage of pain messages to the nervous system and brain.

aromatherapy

For a soothing soak, add 3 drops of lavender, clary sage and Roman chamomile to a warm bath.
Warning Only use clary sage on the day before a period and during the first 2 days of a period.

homeopathy

Lachesis Use this to ease period pains where the flow is very dark and clotted, with cramping pains that move down the thighs as well as radiating to the back.

Colocynthis This can ease rapidly building period pains that come in waves, weakness and faintness resulting from severe pain, and an urge to double-over in an effort to relieve the distress.

Arsenicum album This remedy can ease severe period pains that cause nausea, diarrhoea and/or vomiting, with restlessness and chilliness, and a tendency for severe anxiety.

nutritional approaches

Avoid caffeinated drinks, such as fizzy colas, coffee, tea and chocolate, because caffeine tends to aggravate muscle tension and sensitivity to pain.

naturopathy

• Stimulating the circulation can do much to ease painful periods. Any activity that encourages the large muscles of the legs to move rhythmically, thus increasing the heart and respiration rate, is ideal. Such sustained aerobic exercise promotes the production of endorphins in the body. These 'feel-good' chemicals have natural pain-relieving properties as well as making us feel calmer.

• Applying warmth to the lower abdomen and/or back can be immensely soothing. The simplest way of doing this is to soak in a warm bath. Alternatively, you can apply a towel that has been immersed in warm water and wrung out or a hot-water bottle covered in soft fabric.

western herbalism

Sip a warm infusion of chamomile, lemon balm or lemon verbena to soothe any stress or muscle tension that is contributing to a painful period problem.

heavy periods

This problem can arise at any time during the reproductive years, but there are specific times of life when women are more vulnerable. These include the onset of puberty, when it can take some time for the menstrual cycle to become established, or leading up to the menopause, as the ovaries prepare to stop oestrogen production. Symptoms vary hugely in severity and frequency.

common problems

- **Nausea**
- **Vomiting**
- **Dizziness**
- **Fainting**
- **Uncontrollable, gushing menstrual flow that can soak through even the stoutest form of sanitary protection (such as a tampon plus pad)**
- **Severe cramping pain**
- **Anaemia**

conventional treatments

If there is no apparent reason for the heavy bleeding, your doctor will probably want to examine you to rule out any underlying disorder, such as fibroids, pelvic inflammatory disease or endometriosis. If all seems in order, you may be given medication to control the bleeding.

complementary treatments

These can be especially helpful where the problem is due to hormonal imbalance. While you should consult a trained practitioner if the problem is severe, the following self-help measures may help mild problems of an intermittent nature.

Don't forget that non-conventional medicine can be used in a complementary way, side-by-side with orthodox medical treatment. This can be especially helpful for women approaching the menopause who may find their menstrual cycle has become unpredictable for the first time.

aromatherapy

Add a few drops of geranium, rose or cypress essential oils to a warm bath. These have a reputation for regularizing heavy periods.

homeopathy

Ipecacuanha (Ipecac.) This can ease heavy bleeding that tends to alternate between gushes and steady oozing and is combined with extreme nausea. Both feel much worse for even the slightest movement.

China When periods are very early and so heavy that they trigger problems with vertigo, this remedy may be useful. The bleeding is characteristically very dark and clotted. The severity of blood loss produces faintness and a marked buzzing sensation in the ears.

Lachesis When dreadful cramping pains precede the flow but ease considerably once it starts, consider this remedy. Bleeding can take the form of flooding, with many noticeable large clots in a very dark flow, and may be accompanied by hot flushes and night sweats.

nutritional approaches

• Anaemia may be a complication of heavy bleeding, so include plenty of iron-rich foods in your diet, such as green leafy vegetables, eggs, pulses, oatmeal, molasses, seeds, fish and wholegrain bread. To maximize iron absorption, avoid drinking tea with a meal (this appears to inhibit iron absorption). Instead, take a small glass of orange juice. This can help because vitamin C appears to encourage efficient iron absorption.

• The plant-based oestrogens in soya products also appear to encourage optimum hormone balance. Ring the changes by using soya milk, soya yoghurt, soya cheese and any other foods fortified with soya extract.

western herbalism

If heavy periods seem to be linked to hormonal imbalance, *Agnus castus* may help to restore a healthy balance.

Warning Do not take *Agnus castus* if you are pregnant or if you are taking progesterone drugs or the contraceptive pill, because it may counteract their medicinal action.

irregular periods

The most obvious causes of temporary disruption of a woman's menstrual cycle are pregnancy or the onset of the menopause. However, there are a number of other triggers, which are listed below. Periods can also be naturally irregular at puberty until a regular cycle has been given the chance to establish itself. A severe emotional shock or phase of high stress levels can also disturb the regularity of the menstrual cycle.

common triggers

- **Pregnancy**
- **Onset of the menopause**
- **Anaemia**
- **Eating disorders**
- **Hormone imbalance, including under- or overactive thyroid**
- **Excessive emotional stress over an extended period of time**
- **Excessive exercise, especially when combined with a strict diet**

conventional treatments

A great deal depends on the age and circumstances of the patient. If periods stop suddenly or become erratic when they are normally regular, tests need to be done to rule out pregnancy. A blood test will also be necessary if anaemia or a hormone imbalance is suspected. In women in their late forties, irregular bleeding is usually put down to the onset of the menopause, especially if it is linked to the appearance of hot flushes, poor sleep patterns or night sweats.

complementary treatments

These can be especially helpful in restoring hormonal balance. Once your doctor has established a diagnosis, you should consult an experienced practitioner. Some of the following self-help measures may also be useful.

aromatherapy

Essential oil of rose appears to have hormone-balancing properties. Dilute it in a carrier oil as a massage blend or add or 4 or 5 drops to a warm bath.

relaxation techniques

If it has been decided that this is a stress-related problem, start introducing regular time for relaxation. Studies have shown that the following not only help us to chill out and relax but also may improve our mental focus, concentration and creativity.

- Meditation (including transcendental meditation)
- Autogenic training
- Progressive muscular relaxation (see Yoga, pages 56–57)
- Guided visualization techniques
- Yoga
- Tai chi

prolapse

This problem arises when the ligaments that hold the womb in place lose their elasticity. It is usually related to a series of closely spaced pregnancies. It may also develop after the menopause if the ligaments lose their tone as a result of oestrogen deficiency. A severe prolapse, where the womb protrudes from the vagina, is called a procidentia, but thankfully this is a relatively rare occurrence.

common symptoms

- Collapse of the cervix into the vagina
- A constant sense of pressure or bearing down in the lower abdomen
- An urgent and/or frequent desire to pass water
- Constipation (a severe prolapse may cause or aggravate this)
- Backache
- Stress incontinence

conventional treatments

If pelvic-floor exercises (see below) fail to produce any improvement, it may be necessary to insert a rubber ring to hold up the womb more effectively. This may not be sufficient for a severe prolapse, in which case surgery may be necessary in order to repair the supporting tissues of the womb.

complementary treatments

Any of the following self-help measures can be used alongside conventional treatment.

practicalities

Pelvic-floor exercises (or Kegel exercises) may restore some tone to the muscles of the pelvic floor. These are quite simple to do. Focus on stopping and starting the flow as you pass urine. For maximum benefit do these exercises regularly every day.

homeopathy

Sepia This can ease the negative feelings associated with a mild prolapse caused by closely spaced pregnancies. When the discomfort becomes noticeable, there may be an exhausting feeling of bearing down that can trigger a flatness and depression. When the discomfort is strong, there may also be a marked lowering of libido.

western herbalism

- A mild prolapse may respond to herbs such as raspberry leaf or lady's mantle, which have a reputation for being a uterine tonic.

- A prolapse linked to post-menopausal oestrogen deficiency may respond to a plant-based oestrogen, such as that found in sage.

painful intercourse

This may have a number of causes but the most common is vaginal dryness. A woman may first notice this when she is in her late 40s, especially if the menopause starts early. The problem is that while painful intercourse is unpleasant and life-disrupting enough in itself, lack of moisture in the vagina can increase the risk of infection.

common causes

- **Endometriosis**
- **Vaginitis (inflammation of the vagina and/or vulva)**
- **Vaginismus (spasm of the muscles of the vagina)**
- **Vaginal dryness**
- **Psychological problems**
- **Sexually transmitted diseases**

conventional treatments

These usually involve the application of oestrogen-based creams aimed at restoring the condition of the thinning tissue. If you have an earlier than usual menopause, your doctor may recommend hormone replacement therapy. If there is a psychological cause, he may suggest psycho-sexual counselling. Alternatively, problems with over-tense vaginal muscles that are prone to spasm may respond favourably to specialized physiotherapy exercises.

complementary treatments

Any of the following self-help measures may be helpful and can be used alongside conventional medicines.

practicalities

• If you suffer from recurrent vaginal irritation and inflammation, avoid using scented soaps and foaming bath products. Instead, choose natural products based on essential oils that will usually have a soothing rather than irritating effect.

• It is absolutely essential not to rush foreplay when love-making if you have a tendency to vaginal dryness. If this is not enough, try one of the many lubricating gels available, some of which are based on natural products.

• However tempting it might be to avoid sex, remember that regular orgasms are positively helpful in maintaining the health of the vaginal tissues (as well as being pleasurable for many other reasons!). This is because an orgasm encourages a rush of blood to the genital area. As vaginal dryness can be related to blood flow to the clitoris, vagina, and vulva, which tends to decrease with age, this is obviously beneficial.

aromatherapy

Add a scant few drops of lavender or chamomile essential oils to a warm bath to temporarily ease sensitivity and discomfort.

homeopathy

Sepia This will ease a mild bout of vaginal tenderness that totally reduces the urge to have sex. It is also useful when walking aggravates the itching, irritation and soreness, or where discomfort and unease in the vagina is complicated by a prolapsed womb.

Bryonia When a tendency to vaginal dryness is part of a larger picture of dehydrated mucous membranes, this remedy is more suitable. There may also be a marked tendency to constipation, in which a single large dry stool is passed only with great difficulty. There may also be troublesome burning or irritation in the urinary tract between episodes of passing water.

naturopathy

A soak in a warm bath to which a handful of sea salt has been added can be surprisingly soothing.

western herbalism

• If you are undergoing a particular phase of soreness or inflammation, add a few drops of Calendula or Hypericum tincture to a bidet or warm bath and bathe the affected area.

• If the vulva feels sensitive, apply Calendula cream to soothe and calm the sensitive tissues. Comfrey cream or ointment may serve equally well.

bloating

This uncomfortable and sometimes embarrassing problem is usually related to fluid retention or digestive problems, such as trapped wind or constipation. A classic symptom of bloating tends to be the need to loosen clothing as the day goes on in order to remain comfortable.

common symptoms

- **Tightness around the waistbands of your clothes**
- **The abdomen can feel either soft or hard as a rock, depending on the cause**
- **A lot of rumbling and gurgling, possibly with the passing of wind.**
- **The thighs, ankles and feet may be puffy and swollen, especially if bloating is related to fluid retention (often before the onset of a period)**
- **Constipation**

conventional treatments

If the problem is related to pre-menstrual fluid retention, your doctor may advise you to restrict your salt intake, as well as prescribing a short-term course of diuretic (fluid-eliminating) drugs. If digestive problems seem to be the more likely cause, you may be advised on the best ways of achieving and maintaining regular bowel movements.

complementary treatments

Like conventional doctors, a conventional therapist's first aim is to establish the cause of the problem. Severe and/or well-established problems of bloating respond best to professional complementary treatment. However, the following self-help measures may be of use in treating milder or more low-level bloating.

nutritional approaches

• Try eliminating wheat products from your diet, to see whether the symptoms improve. Try this for a month, substituting bread with rice cakes (these soothe and regulate the digestive system and encourage the smooth working of the bowel). If you miss the texture of wheat breads, try a light rye variety instead. If your symptoms improve, but return if you introduce wheat products, you may be sensitive to wheat. If this is the case, you should consult a nutritional therapist.

• If fluid retention is a problem, try regulating your salt intake. Watch out for pre-menstrual cravings for salty snacks, such as crisps and nuts, which may make the problem worse. Eat plenty of fresh, leafy green vegetables to boost your potassium intake and thus maintain a healthy balance of sodium and potassium. Watch out for hidden sources of sodium, such as monosodium glutamate in Chinese dishes.

naturopathy

• If bloating is definitely due to sluggish digestion, becoming more physically active will greatly help the situation. This has the double effect of toning up the muscles of the abdomen and making the bowels work more smoothly and efficiently.

• Drinking plenty of water every day will also help. However, be sure to drink only still mineral water or filtered tap water. This is especially important where bloating is concerned because fizzy waters can aggravate the symptoms.

• Pilates or yoga can be useful for toning the abdomen.

homeopathy

Lycopodium This can help abdominal bloating that's accompanied by lots of rumbling and gurgling sounds. It can also help regulate bowel movements that may alternate between diarrhoea and constipation as a result of temporarily high stress levels.

Apis This can encourage the elimination of excess fluid around the abdomen or ankles that may be especially noticeable pre-menstrually. The breasts may also feel enlarged and water-logged before a period.

breast pain

Breast tissue is immensely sensitive and subject to constant periodic changes. Tenderness or enlargement are a natural part of the menstrual cycle and are quite familiar to most of us. Most changes are temporary and commonly occur before a period or during the menopause. However, if you notice any unusual changes, you should seek medical advice.

common symptoms

- Pain on touching the breasts or from the slightest movement or pressure (such as turning over in bed or running down stairs).
- Enlargement of the breasts before a period, perhaps by a whole cup size
- Intensely sensitive and reactive nipples

warning symptoms

- A discernible lump or mass of tissue
- Any noticeable puckering of skin or indentation
- Discharge from either nipple
- Enlarged or tender glands in the armpit

conventional treatments

The first stage usually involves a manual examination and perhaps a mammogram (X-ray of the breast). If a lump is found, you may be given a needle biopsy to determine whether or not it is malignant. If it is malignant, treatment usually involves chemotherapy, radiotherapy and/or surgery. If one or more cysts are present, they may be drained by a technique known as aspiration.

complementary treatments

Any of the following can help ease very mild breast pain that is obviously linked to hormonal fluctuations leading up to a period. Any other problems with breast pain that are unusual, severe or well established should be diagnosed and treated by a trained practitioner of complementary medicine.

aromatherapy

When your breasts are tender, add a few drops of geranium, juniper, rosemary and lavender essential oils to your bathwater to gently encourage efficient lymphatic drainage and help hormonal balance.

homeopathy

Bryonia Breast pain that is made significantly worse by the slightest movement and eased by keeping still may respond to this remedy.

Lachesis This is specifically for breast pain that sets in at ovulation and builds up until the period starts, when it disappears immediately.

nutritional approaches

• If you have occasional period-related breast pain, cut down or avoid coffee, other caffeinated drinks and dairy products (both can aggravate the development of breast cysts, and both are difficult for the lymphatic system to eliminate).

• Take oil of evening primrose supplements to help benign breast pain and swelling.

naturopathy

A simple hydrotherapy technique will tone up the breasts generally. It requires no more than a couple of bowls, one of warm water and one of cold, and a couple of flannels. Soak one flannel in hot water, wring it out and apply it to each breast in turn. Follow this with a flannel that has been soaked in cold water. Repeat this routine three times, being sure to finish with the cold flannel.

western herbalism

If period-related breast tenderness is associated with fluid retention, try dandelion tea which is thought to encourage the elimination of excess fluid.

thrush

Thrush is due to an overgrowth of a yeast (a type of fungus) called *Candida albicans*. This is present in everyone's gut and is normally kept in check. However, if the healthy balance of the body is disturbed, it can spread from the gut into the vagina, giving rise to the symptoms of thrush. Thrush can also cause symptoms in the mouth, or on the skin, especially under the breasts.

common symptoms

- **Vaginal itching and irritation**
- **Thick, white, cheesy discharge**
- **An increasingly frequent and urgent need to pass water**
- **Soreness and burning when passing water**
- **Painful intercourse**

conventional treatments

Treatment Involves anti-fungal medication in the form of a cream that is applied to the affected area and a pessary that is inserted into the vagina. Alternatively, a single tablet may be taken by mouth.

complementary treatments

Any of the measures given below will be helpful in easing a single, mild bout of thrush and all can be used alongside conventional treatment. For more established thrush problems you should consult an experienced practitioner.

Nutritional medicine in particular has a great deal to offer in the way of managing and ultimately eliminating a case of well-established candida overgrowth.

practicalities

• Avoid highly scented bath products, which can aggravate thrush symptoms. Try a soothing salt-water bath instead.

• Wearing tights or close-fitting jeans during an acute episode of thrush creates exactly the sort of warm, moist environment that Candida loves. Instead, wear stockings rather than tights, underwear made from natural fibres such as cotton or silk, and a skirt or loose-fitting trousers.

• Do not use creams that have a temporary anaesthetizing effect. These may suppress itching in the short-term but can trigger further sensitivity.

• If you have been taking antibiotics, eat live yoghurt to re-establish the healthy bacteria in the gut.

aromatherapy

Add 10 drops of lavender essential oil to a warm bath for a soothing, irritation-relieving soak.

homeopathy

Natrum muriaticum (Nat mur.) This may be helpful where thrush is accompanied by a vaginal discharge that is either thin, clear and watery or jelly-like (like raw egg white). The vagina may also feel dry and sore.

Borax Bouts of thrush that occur specifically at ovulation (mid-cycle) may be soothed by this remedy. The vagina is likely to feel irritated, sore and swollen, with a strange sensation of warm water flowing down the thighs.

Pulsatilla Thrush problems dating from pregnancy or the onset of regular periods may be eased by this. Vaginal discharges may be thick and yellowish, and any general irritation and discomfort is worsened by getting over-heated.

nutritional approaches

• Avoid sugar in any form, cheese, pickles and mushrooms, and foods produced by fermentation, such as alcohol and bread, all of which have been linked to Candida overgrowth.

• Choose unrefined wholefoods, especially items such as garlic and bio-yoghurt which appear to support the healthy balance of gut microorganisms.

• Apply cool natural bio-yoghurt to the irritated area. If this is messy, use a panty liner to protect your clothes.

western herbalism

• Add this infusion to your bathwater for a soothing soak.

Add 1 teaspoonful of dried marigold, golden seal, rosemary, thyme or fennel to a cup of boiling water and leave to infuse for 15 minutes before straining.

Warning Do not use golden seal or rosemary during pregnancy.

• *Take Echinacea internally for the duration of the symptoms to support your immune system's fight against infection.*

morning sickness

This nausea and vomiting is by no means inevitable in the first 3 months or so of pregnancy, but it can be distressing when it sets in with regularity and severity. An unfortunate minority of women suffer from it throughout their pregnancy, while others find that it persists throughout the day. Common symptoms, which occur in varying degrees of severity, are listed below.

common symptoms

- **Severe nausea triggered or made worse by exposure to the sight or smell of food**
- **Vomiting or gagging**
- **Dizziness**
- **Weariness**

conventional treatments

Treatment of mild to moderate morning sickness usually consists of advice about practical lifestyle changes that can ease some of the symptoms (see Naturopathy and Nutritional approaches opposite). Where vomiting is severe and frequent, hospital admission may be necessary to deal with the risk of dehydration.

complementary treatments

Any of the following self-help measures may be used in the short term to relieve mild to moderate morning sickness. However, for more severe problems, you should consult an experienced practitioner.

Since high stress levels appear to aggravate symptoms of morning sickness and nausea, it's worth considering taking up any activity that you find especially relaxing.

acupressure

Studies show that the acupressure bands worn on the wrist to prevent travel sickness also reduce nausea in pregnant women.

homeopathy

Pulsatilla Morning sickness that lasts all day and evening may respond to this remedy, especially if there is a marked aversion to fatty foods, such as creamy sauces or meats that are difficult to digest, such as pork. Despite feelings of chilliness, being in overly hot, stuffy surroundings is likely to make the nausea worse.

Sepia Nausea and vomiting that are triggered or made noticeably worse by the thought, sight or smell of food will do better with Sepia. This remedy is especially indicated where a noticeably drained, exhausted mood alternates between indifference, irritability and depression.

Nux vomica This may ease morning sickness that feels hugely relieved after vomiting, although it can be very difficult to bring up the food, with much gagging, straining and retching being necessary. It is also helpful in reducing stress and tension in the early stages of pregnancy.

nutritional approaches

It is interesting that pregnant women (especially in the early months) often develop an aversion to the foods and drinks that make nausea worse. These include dairy foods or other items high in fat, strong tea, coffee, alcohol and cigarettes. In any case, they should all be avoided.

naturopathy

If nausea and vomiting start as soon as you get up or even sit up in the morning, keep a plain biscuit and a glass of water beside your bed. Eating something as soon as you wake will help to prevent nausea. This is because low blood sugar levels, common on waking, can aggravate feelings of sickness. For the same reason, eating regular small quantities of something light and nutritious every couple of hours will keep your blood sugar levels stable.

western herbalism

Sipping a warm infusion of chamomile, peppermint or lemon balm tea can help soothe a queasy stomach.

recovery after childbirth

This is one area where complementary approaches to healing can offer a huge amount of help and support. This is good news, since even the most positive experience of labour and delivery can put an enormous strain on the mother's body. As a result, both physical and emotional recovery can take a little while. Within this context, complementary therapies will speed up the process that would eventually happen naturally.

common problems

- **Exhaustion and fatigue**
- **Pain associated with an episiotomy or stitches that are slow to heal**
- **Internal bruising**
- **Restricted movement, such as lifting or driving after a Caesarian**
- **Emotional issues, perhaps if a hoped-for natural birth fails to go to plan and more intrusive measures or a Caesarian are necessary**

conventional treatments

This tends to involve making sure that stitches are healing well and free of infection, and advice about activities (such as driving and lifting heavy weights) that need to be treated with caution, especially after a Caesarian.

complementary treatments

Any of the following measures can be used alongside conventional treatments. Complementary treatments offer the huge advantage of providing support to both mind and body when stimulating a fast, effective recovery. For instance, the homeopathic remedy Arnica helps as much with the psychological effects of shock as it does with physical trauma.

aromatherapy

If after-pains are a problem (these may be especially strong when starting to breastfeed), add a few drops of chamomile, lavender or marjoram essential oils to your bath. These antispasmodic oils are very soothing. Alternatively, holding a warm compress of these essential oils to the abdomen may do the trick.

homeopathy

Arnica This is the first remedy to turn to after labour and delivery largely because of its ability to support the system while it rebalances itself after a challenging or traumatic time.

China Use this to lift exhaustion that is related directly to blood loss and takes the form of extreme irritability and being on an extremely short emotional and mental fuse.

Kalium phosphoricum (Kali phos.) This helps lift the tiredness and exhaustion resulting from the disturbance of a regular sleep pattern by the demands of a newborn who has yet to get into a routine. Symptoms include nervousness, anxiety and difficulty in mentally focusing on anything taxing or demanding.

Sepia In the first few days after the birth, this can be incredibly helpful in lifting the feelings of emotional flatness and exhaustion associated with hormonal imbalance.

Pulsatilla In the days immediately after the birth, this can relieve any persistent weepiness, which may start to be exhausting, as well as helping general mood swings that are connected to hormonal imbalance.

western herbalism

Add a few drops of diluted Calendula tincture to a warm bath or bidet and bathe the perineal area. Alternatively, dilute 1 part tincture to 10 parts water, apply to a sanitary towel and hold it over the perineum. This is immensely soothing and speeds up the healing of tissue. A formula that also contains Hypericum will provide natural pain relief as well.

bach flower remedies

Olive can reduce the general fatigue and physical, mental and emotional exhaustion that make it so hard to cope with the daily demands of a new baby. Tiredness may reach such a level that it feels impossible to go on.

Olive can be taken by making up a treatment bottle. Fill a 28g (1oz) dropper bottle with filtered or still mineral water and add two drops of the flower remedy plus a teaspoon of brandy to preserve the solution. Take four drops in a small glass of water four times a day.

painful stitches

Stitches are not inevitable after delivery, unless there has been a tear in the perineum or an episiotomy. Also, in the case of a Caesarian, stitches or clips are necessary to hold the abdominal wound together long enough for healing to take place. Effective complementary treatment can encourage fast granulation of tissue so that the wound can heal speedily.

common causes

- **A fast labour**
- **Need for forceps or Venteuse delivery**

common symptoms

- **Tenderness and sensitivity of the area that has been stitched, even for some time after healing has taken place.**

conventional treatments

This tends to involve regular checks to see that healing is progressing well, the wound looks healthy, and that there are no signs of infection. Bathing the affected parts in salty water may be advised.

complementary treatments

These can be used alongside conventional measures as a means of speeding up the healing process and reducing pain and discomfort.

western herbalism

- Ease the pain of recently stitched areas by bathing them in warm water to which a dilute solution of combined Calendula and Hypericum tincture has been added. Calendula acts as a natural antiseptic and promotes fast healing of lacerated tissue, while Hypericum reduces pain.

- Once the wounds have healed, massage comfrey ointment gently into the area to reduce the possibility of scarring.

aromatherapy

Add a few drops of chamomile, cypress or lavender essential oils to a warm bath or bidet and bathe the affected parts. This will encourage the damaged tissues to heal as efficiently as possible and soothe general discomfort.

homeopathy

Arnica Given initially, this helps with the general trauma that follows birth, whether natural or by Caesarian.

Staphysagria This eases the pain and sensitivity of areas that have been stitched. It can also help some of the negative emotions that accompany a high-tech birth, such as disappointment, resentment and unexpressed anger, which can manifest as depression and extreme emotional sensitivity.

internal bruising

Even the most straightforward labour and delivery involve some degree of internal bruising and trauma of the birth canal, and this can take a while to settle down. The situation is exacerbated if there have been any complications, and under these circumstances complementary medical support is going to be of value in speeding up healing.

common causes

- **Complications entailing invasive intervention**
- **Use of forceps**
- **Venteuse delivery**
- **Unexpectedly sudden and quick birth**

conventional treatments

This usually consists of checking that healing is progressing well and making sure that there are no signs of infection.

complementary treatments

The following measures can be of immense practical help and support in gently and naturally encouraging re-absorption of blood, and easing the pain and sensitivity of traumatized tissues.

homeopathy

Arnica This is the first remedy to use for internal bruising, since it is noted for stimulating the efficient re-absorption of blood from bruised areas and reducing swelling and discomfort.

Bellis perennis This can be given after Arnica has improved, but not fully resolved, fairly extensive or severe bruising.

western herbalism

Bathe as soon as possible in a diluted tincture of Hypericum to soothe pain and discomfort in the delicate tissues of the perineum that are rich in nerves.

sore nipples

When we consider their incredible sensitivity, it is not surprising that the pain and discomfort of sore, cracked nipples are so unbearable. Unfortunately, once established, this problem can make breastfeeding very difficult or impossible, making the mother tense and unhappy. When this happens, a negative cycle can be set up that leaves both mother and baby very distressed.

common causes

- **The baby is not latching on to the nipple well enough when breastfeeding**
- **Thrush (if your baby has oral thrush)**

conventional treatments

If you are finding breastfeeding really difficult, and if your baby prefers to 'graze' or snack frequently, rather than taking a complete feed when put to the breast, ask your health visitor for advice. If only one breast is affected, applying a soothing cream to the breast for a few days may help the nipple to heal.

complementary treatments

Any of the practical measures listed below will help to prevent the nipples becoming painful. They will also lessen the risk of cracking, which is especially important because any obvious breaks in the skin can lead to infection and possibly mastitis (pages 186–87).

practicalities

Encouraging your baby to feed correctly is essential if you want to reduce the risk of developing painful nipples.

• Make sure that your baby is positioned properly, so that he or she takes both the nipple and the surrounding area (the areola) into the mouth.

• If your baby is in the optimum position for feeding, the nipple should be well into the mouth so that the tongue is used effectively for suckling.

• Before taking your baby from the breast, put your finger gently into his or her mouth in order to break the contact between mouth and nipple. This will help prevent further damage to the nipple.

• Between feeds, wear nipple shields inside your brassiere. These allow air to circulate, so that the nipples are kept as dry as possible.

aromatherapy

Add a few drops of rose essential oil to a carrier oil and massage gently into the sore areas. Wash off the oil thoroughly before the next feed.

homeopathy

Graphites This is almost a specific for severely cracked, painfully sensitive nipples. The left breast may be more affected than the right, and discomfort is often more noticeable at night, resulting in tiredness and fatigue during the day.

western herbalism

• Bathe your nipples with a 1 in 10 dilution of Hypericum and Calendula tincture between feeds. Then apply Calendula cream liberally to the sore areas, being sure to wipe the nipple with a soft, moist cloth before your baby begins feeding again. After feeding, be sure to bathe the nipples and reapply the cream.

• Apply comfrey ointment to soothe sore tissues and encourage speedy healing. Always make sure to remove any traces of the ointment before your baby's next feed.

mastitis

This painful condition sets in when a duct in the breast becomes blocked, resulting in the formation of a breast abscess. Alternatively, it may result from an infection of cracked nipples. The symptoms, which are fairly unmistakable, are listed below.

Warning Once you reach the late stage, you should seek medical attention promptly.

common symptoms

Early stage

- **Lumpiness, pain and discomfort in the affected breast**
- **Inflammation, heat and redness of the skin immediately above the affected area**

Late stage

- **A high temperature and general feeling of unwellness**

conventional treatments

If a breast examination shows that infection has set in, your doctor will probably prescribe a course of antibiotics.

complementary treatments

In the early stages, any of the following measures may prevent the situation from progressing to the point where an infection develops. However, once you start to run a high temperature and feel generally unwell, you should consult your doctor as soon as possible.

practicalities

• Make sure that your breasts do not become engorged with milk because this will make you more vulnerable to mastitis. If you cannot persuade your baby to feed regularly, use a breast pump between feeds to stop your breasts feeling over-full and painful.

• Keep up your fluid intake by drinking glasses of still mineral water or filtered tap water regularly.

• Massage your breasts gently but firmly between feeds to stimulate the circulation.

• Try to make sure that each breast is drained as fully as possible at every feed. It helps if you position your baby so that any potential blockage is drained by the force of gravity.

• Make sure that your maternity bra is not too tight or constricting.

aromatherapy

Add a few drops of chamomile, rose or lavender essential oils to a bowl of warm water, immerse a clean flannel in the water, wring it out and apply it as a warm compress to the affected breast.

homeopathy

Bryonia Breast pain that is extremely sensitive to the slightest movement and eased by keeping as still as possible and applying firm pressure to the painful area may respond to this remedy. Breasts may feel very hard and over-sensitive as a result of low-level dehydration.

Phytolacca This can relieve breast tenderness that involves general aching, sore, sensitive glands, shooting pains radiating from the affected breast to the armpit, and sore, sensitive or cracked nipples.

Belladonna This can be very helpful in reducing a fast-developing inflammation if it is caught at the earliest stage. The affected area of the breast may become extremely painful, hot and red very quickly, possibly with red streaks radiating from the nipple. Pain and discomfort is made more intense by jarring movement, lying flat in bed and/or being touched.

naturopathy

Apply warm and cold flannels alternately to the affected breast (see also Breast pain, pages 174–75).

polycystic ovary syndrome

This distressing chronic condition, also referred to as PCOS, can produce a wide range of unpleasant symptoms, differing in combination and severity. It may also affect fertility. Because of the hormone imbalance, the body produces an excessive amount of androgene that plays a large part in the production of male symptoms, such as excessive body hair.

common symptoms

- **Weight gain**
- **Irregular periods or cessation of periods**
- **Excess body and facial hair**
- **Extreme tiredness and exhaustion**
- **Difficulty in conceiving**
- **An increased risk of developing Type 2 diabetes and/or heart disease**
- **Skin problems, including acne**
- **Mood swings**

conventional treatments

Treatment aims to control the symptoms as far as possible with hormonal drugs (such as the contraceptive pill or androgen suppressants). If you are anxious to conceive, you may be given short-term medication designed to induce ovulation.

complementary treatments

Because of the chronic nature of this condition and the range of potentially debilitating symptoms that may accompany it, you should consult a skilled practitioner of complementary medicine. Most practitioners will focus on restoring a healthy balance in the whole system and factors that are known to aggravate PCOS, such as being significantly overweight. The following measures may be of help and can be used alongside conventional treatment.

practicalities

For healthy weight loss, it is important to combine dietary improvements with a regular exercise programme. Whatever system of fitness you choose be sure that you can commit yourself to a regular routine. This is important because four 35-minute sessions a week will be much more effective in helping you reach your target weight than one 2-hour session of frenetic activity a week.

nutritional approaches

• Keep your blood sugar levels, and therefore your energy levels, stable by avoiding the sugar 'rush' that comes from eating items made from refined white sugar (including sweetened drinks, such as fizzy colas, and sauces and ketchups, which all contain large amounts of 'hidden' sugar). It also helps to eat something every couple of hours (ideally a piece of fruit, fresh, raw chunks of vegetables or a rice cake made from organic brown rice with a savoury topping). Recent research has confirmed that regular cups of coffee raise our blood sugar levels, even if it is black with no sugar.

• Eat dairy products in moderation because they are thought to aggravate hormonal imbalance. Instead, opt for foods that are natural sources of plant-based oestrogens, such as tofu and pulses.

naturopathy

Loss of excess weight should be a top priority because being significantly overweight increases the levels of androgens (male hormones that aggravate symptoms such as hair growth). It also increases the risk of complications such as Type 2 diabetes and heart disease. Avoid crash diets (especially low-calorie or low-fat diets) because these do little to improve our nutritional status. Instead, eat regular small amounts of unrefined carbohydrates (such as wholegrains), fish, fresh fruit, crisp vegetables and moderate amounts of dairy foods.

endometriosis

This distressing condition affects women from their late 20s to the end of their fertile years. It is caused by a proliferation of endometrial tissue (the lining of the womb) into areas such as the ovaries or inside the muscle of the womb. These tissues bleed during a period, but because there is no outlet for the blood, there may be very severe pain. Certain factors appear to increase the risk of endometriosis.

common symptoms

- **Excruciatingly painful periods**
- **Painful intercourse**
- **Fluid retention**
- **Weight gain**
- **Breast tenderness**
- **Infertility**

common triggers

- **Delayed first pregnancy**
- **Late onset of puberty**
- **Excessive oestrogen production**
- **High levels of stress**

conventional treatments

Diagnosis is usually by a laparoscopy, which entails inserting a tiny camera into the abdomen. Treatment may involve prescription drugs designed to inhibit ovulation. Alternatively, if the condition is not too widespread, it may be possible to surgically remove the pockets of endometriosis. The last resort, if problems are very severe and widespread, is a hysterectomy.

complementary treatments

Complementary therapies have a significant track record in helping patients with endometriosis, by reducing pain and possibly preventing the condition from escalating. However, this is a chronic condition, it must be treated by an experienced practitioner and self-help is not really an option.

therapies to consider

If you wish to consult a trained practitioner, consider one of the following:

- Eastern therapies
- Chinese herbalism
- Natural therapies
- Homeopathy
- Naturopathy
- Nutritional therapy
- Western herbalism

homeopathy

These are some of the possibilities that a practitioner may consider.

Lachesis For symptoms that build with progressive intensity from mid-cycle to the beginning of a period, left-sided ovarian pain may be marked, while the blood during a period may be dark and clotted. Mood swings are also very noticeable before a period, lifting as soon as the bleed is established.

Sepia This can help the sense of profound emotional, mental and physical exhaustion that can descend before a period. Bearing down sensations occur with severe menstrual cramps: this may or may not be exaggerated by the existence of a prolapse as a result of pregnancies that have occurred with little time gap in between.

Nux vomica This can help ease painful periods that are due to high levels of stress and tension that may exaggerate menstrual cramps. Symptoms are made noticeably worse by a high coffee intake and feeling irritable and under pressure.

aromatherapy

Add a few drops of lavender, chamomile or marjoram and/or rosemary essential oils to a warm bath in order to soothe abdominal cramps.

infertility

The inability to conceive affects about one in ten couples in the Western world. When a baby is desperately wanted, this can be a very stressful and distressing situation for both partners. There are a number of possible obstacles to conception and these are listed below. Ironically, being under stress can itself be a major co-factor in making conception difficult.

causes (female)

- **Blocked fallopian tubes**
- **Abnormalities with cervical mucus**
- **Structural problems of the womb**
- **Low progesterone levels**
- **Ovulation problems**
- **Endometriosis**
- **Stress**

causes (male)

- **A low sperm count**
- **Sperm irregularity with low motility (rate of movement)**
- **Problems with ejaculation, including premature ejaculation**

conventional treatments

If a couple have been unsuccessfully trying to conceive for 2 years, each partner will probably be given a series of tests to establish the nature of the problem. These usually involve blood tests, ultra-sound scans and/or a laparoscopy. Drugs may be given to stimulate ovulation and, finally, IVF (in vitro fertilization) may be considered an option.

counselling

Counselling may be helpful where one or both partners have difficulty in expressing their anxieties. This provides the couple with a safe space in which to acknowledge, explore and resolve their feelings.

complementary treatments

If both partners have been tested and there appears to be no obvious reason for the failure to conceive, complementary treatments can be especially helpful. These are most successful if given by a trained practitioner, but the self-help measures given below are worth following if conception is desired.

practicalities

Knowing when they are at their most fertile is a priority for women who wish to conceive. For women with a regular 28-day cycle, this is most likely to be on days 13, 14 and 15. Useful signs to look for include a change in the consistency of vaginal mucus (it becomes much more liquid and jelly-like at this time). Alternatively, using an ovulation kit can take some of the guesswork out of the situation.

ayurveda

Garlic, onion and asparagus are among the foods thought to increase fertility.

aromatherapy

Add a few drops of essential oils of rose, geranium and melissa to a warm bath, or dilute them in a carrier oil and massage them over the abdominal area daily.

nutritional approaches

Avoid alcohol, convenience foods, caffeine and red meat, which all have a negative affect on fertility. Foods with a positive effect include the essential fatty acids found in seeds, nuts and oily fish. Dietary supplements of folic acid and vitamin B6 may be helpful.

naturopathy

If fertility is an issue, giving up smoking is a priority for both partners. In women, smoking appears to have an adverse effect on the blood flow to the neck of the womb and on the action of the cilia (fine hairs) that guide the egg down the oviduct to the womb. In men (according to a recent report in the *British Medical Journal*), smoking reduces the blood flow to the genital area and reduces both the quality and mobility of semen.

western herbalism

If a hormone imbalance is suspected (for instance, after a few years of taking a contraceptive pill), hormone-balancing herbs may be helpful. Possibilities include *Agnus castus* and false unicorn root. Ideally, these should be administered by a trained practitioner, who will establish the optimum dosage. They must be discontinued once conception has been confirmed.

hypnotherapy

Excessive stress can play a significant role in reducing the chances of conception. Research from the Chelsea and Westminster Hospital in London in the mid-1990s showed that hypnotherapy was successful in helping conception by reducing stress levels.

early menopause

The menopause is when periods finally stop; it may occur at any age between the mid-40s and the mid-50s, the average being 51. A much earlier menopause is a cause for concern because health problems such as osteoporosis (low bone density) and an increased risk of heart disease can develop. Common triggers of an early menopause and menopausal symptoms, which vary in range and severity, are listed below.

common symptoms

- Hot flushes and night sweats
- Insomnia
- Mood swings
- Erratic and heavy periods
- Fatigue

common triggers

- Surgery involving removal of the womb and/or ovaries
- Cancer treatments, such as chemotherapy and/or radiotherapy
- Low body weight, especially if there is a history of strict dieting or eating disorders
- Poor diet combined with heavy smoking and/or alcohol intake
- Addiction to exercise that has contributed to a very low body weight

conventional treatments

The earlier the menopause, the greater the risk of osteoporosis. Hormone replacement therapy (HRT) was the first resort until concerns were raised about the safety of its long-term use. It is now no longer regarded as the most appropriate treatment and is being replaced with drugs that are targeted at improving bone density. Short-term use of HRT is still thought appropriate for severe hot flushes and night sweats.

complementary treatments

These can help enormously, either alone or combined with conventional treatment. Unlike conventional doctors, who tend to view menopause in terms of oestrogen deficiency, complementary practitioners regard menopause as a natural rite of passage that needs appropriate support so that it can be accomplished as smoothly and efficiently as possible.

practicalities

• Take regular, weight-bearing, rhythmic exercise to protect and maintain healthy bone density. Studies of women who took a brisk walk four times a week showed an increase in the bone density of the spine of up to 5 per cent, whereas women who took no exercise lost 7 per cent of this bone density.

• Regular exercise can also help to improve body confidence by creating a stronger, leaner body, as well as helping to regulate and balance energy levels, which are known to flag at menopause.

homeopathy

Sepia This can help manage hot flushes, fatigue and low mood associated with an early menopause. It can also be helpful in boosting a flagging libido.

Lachesis This can help restore a sound sleep pattern that's been disturbed by frequent, drenching night sweats. It can also help rebalance mood swings that shift from 'hyper' to low very quickly.

nutritional approaches

• A sound nutritional approach can play a central role in protecting us from some of the complications of early menopause. Make sure that you have a healthy calcium intake in order to maintain bone density. Remember that there are other sources of this mineral apart from dairy foods, such as dark green vegetables, tofu, seeds, oily fish (such as salmon or sardines) and unsalted nuts.

• Magnesium and vitamin D are also essential for efficient calcium absorption. Obtain these from seafood, apples, seaweed, tofu, sesame seeds, fish and fish oils.

• Smoking and a high alcohol intake may also encourage an early menopause, especially if combined with any of the triggers listed above. Both habits lower oestrogen production and increase the risk of osteoporosis.

weight gain

Nowadays, the issue of what constitutes a healthy weight seems to be full of contradictions and confusion. What is popularly regarded as a desirable weight often differs significantly from a realistic healthy weight, and it is important to distinguish between the two. The guidelines listed below should help you to establish whether or not your weight is at a healthy level.

are you over-weight?

- **Do you get breathless climbing a moderate flight of stairs or walking at a moderate pace?**
- **Do you get out of breath after running a short distance?**
- **Are there obvious signs of excess weight on your upper arms, thighs or belly?**
- **Does your clothing feel uncomfortably tight after a short period of time?**

If you answer 'yes' to all of the questions, you might seek advice on how best to lose a few pounds. However, if you answer 'no', you may still be a reasonably healthy weight for your build.

conventional treatments

Weight gain may be related to an under-active thyroid gland, in which case you may be given medication to restore your thyroxine levels. If there is no obvious underlying condition contributing to weight gain, you may be given advice about diet and exercise plans.

complementary treatments

Any of the following measures will help you to achieve and maintain a healthy weight. Do bear in mind that what you should be striving for is long-term stability at a healthy weight, rather than attempting to go on a drastic diet to reach an unrealistic dress size. As a basic rule of thumb, the faster the weight comes off, the faster it's likely to go back on.

practicalities

At all costs, avoid crash diets. Not only are many of these highly suspect nutritionally, because they are so unbalanced, but they also programme our bodies to gain weight as soon as we resume normal eating. Moreover, crash dieting increases the chance of developing cellulite on the upper arms, belly and thighs.

nutritional approaches

• A simple and effective way of establishing whether you are over-eating or eating unhealthy foods is to list everything that you eat and drink for 2 or 3 days. You must include every nibble and snack for this to be truly helpful. You may be amazed at the results!

• Remember that the foods and drinks that tend to make us gain weight are usually those that are nutritionally deficient. Such foods include white rice and items containing large amounts of white sugar and white flour, additives, colourings and preservatives (like sodium). Instead, opt for healthier alternatives, such as wholegrain cereals, unrefined rice, vegetables, fruit and small amounts of dairy foods, and always drink plenty of water. These items are more likely to keep hunger pangs at bay, thus making it less likely that you will over-eat.

• Avoid high-fat, highly processed foods because the hydrogenated fats that they contain can contribute to hormone imbalance. Also avoid items advertised as being low fat, which are often high in sugar and/or artificial sweeteners. Instead, opt for high-fibre foods that are as natural as possible, such as generous portions of fresh vegetables, home-made soups, pulses, wholegrain cereals and unsalted nuts and seeds.

pilates and yoga

• Regular exercise not only helps build stronger and more supple muscles, but systems of movement such as Pilates and yoga encourage the development of a leaner, more slender body while sacrificing absolutely nothing in the fitness stakes.

• As a healthy bonus, you may find that regular exercise decreases your appetite naturally rather than increasing it.

hot flushes

These are one of the most common features of the menopause, and about 70 per cent of pre-menopausal and menopausal women report having hot flushes to some degree. They appear to be triggered by the rapid decline in the amount of oestrogen secreted by the ovaries as the menopause begins, and they vary in severity and frequency.

common features

- Abrupt onset of waves of heat that wash over the body, sometimes followed by drenching perspiration
- A sense of panic or vague unease before a hot flush
- Pronounced reddening of the skin on the affected areas of the body, usually the neck, face and chest

conventional treatments

Until recently, hot flushes were usually treated with hormone replacement therapy (HRT). However, a study conducted by the Women's Health Initiative in the United States raised sufficient safety concerns to stop further trials. As a result, the indications are that HRT should be used for as short a time as possible.

complementary treatments

For women who want an effective treatment for hot flushes without the side-effects of HRT, these offer very positive benefits. Given the negative publicity associated with HRT, it could be persuasively argued that complementary therapies should be the first resort for women who have classic hot flushes.

practicalities

• Since hot flushes are the result of the body's thermostat going hay-wire (making us unable to adapt quickly and effectively to temperature changes), it makes sense to dress appropriately. For example, if you wear a loose, short-sleeved top with a jacket or cardigan, it is easy to remove the top layer when your temperature rises.

• Wear clothes made from natural fibres, such as cotton, linen or silk, which absorb perspiration and allow the body to cool down more effectively. Avoid clothes made from synthetic fabrics or microfibres, which keep in the heat and perspiration and prevent the skin from cooling down.

• Regular aerobic exercise can help if hot flushes are a noticeable or frequent problem. Consider walking, gentle jogging or 'power walking', cycling or swimming.

aromatherapy

To relieve mild, infrequent hot flushes. add a scant few drops of clary sage or cypress essential oils to a warm (not hot) bath a couple of hours before retiring. Hot water is not only generally enervating but may also trigger hot flushes.

homeopathy

Lachesis This is very helpful in relieving hot flushes that occur with distressing regularity on waking. Any constriction around the throat, such as a high-necked jumper or a scarf, can feel suffocating.

Sepia Try this remedy to relieve flushes that are accompanied by feeling mentally, emotionally and physically drained. Flushes that occur regularly can be exhausting, triggering emotional flatness or depression.

Calcarea carbonica (Calc. carb.) This remedy can help when hot flushes are followed by drenching, clammy perspiration, especially if they are triggered by the slightest physical effort and a general sense of the whole system becoming slower and more sluggish.

nutritional approaches

• To keep hot flushes at bay, eat plenty of foods that are rich in plant-based oestrogens. These oestrogens are found in soya-based products, such as tofu and soya milk, and appear to buffer the decline in oestrogen secretion at menopause. It is interesting to note that, in the Far East, where soya products form a major part of the diet, hot flushes are not considered a problem.

• Certain foods and drinks are thought to aggravate hot flushes, such as alcohol, caffeinated drinks (including tea and colas, as well as coffee) and spicy foods.

night sweats

These are the nocturnal version of hot flushes and can occur at any time in the years leading up to and including the menopause. Symptoms vary in intensity and can include any combination of those listed below.

common features

- **Difficulty in switching off and falling asleep because of raised body temperature**
- **Drifting off to sleep easily, but waking during the night in a sweat**
- **Sweats just before getting up in the morning**
- **Severe sweats that can force you out of bed**

conventional treatments

The usual treatment for night sweats used to be hormone replacement therapy (HRT). However, recent studies have raised safety concerns about this treatment (see Hot Flushes, pages 198–99). As a result, some conventional doctors may suggest that complementary medical treatment should be the first port of call. If this isn't appropriate for any reason, they may suggest opting for treatment with HRT for the minimal amount of time in order to reduce the scale and severity of the problem.

complementary treatments

Given the concerns about hormone replacement therapy, the benefits of complementary therapies are very attractive.

practicalities

• Take steps to pre-empt the problem. Keep a bowl of tepid water, a sponge or flannel, a towel and a change of nightwear beside your bed. If you wake, a quick sponge-down and a change of nightwear will give you a good chance of getting back to sleep again.

• Keep your bedroom well-ventilated but not so cold that you end up feeling chilly when sweating has reached the clammy stage.

• Choose bed linen and nightwear made from natural fibres, which allow the skin to breathe, rather than synthetic fabrics (see also Hot flushes, pages 198–99).

• Regular exercise that stimulates the circulation can help if night sweats are a noticeable or frequent problem. Consider walking, gentle jogging or 'power walking', cycling or swimming.

aromatherapy

To relieve mild, infrequent night sweats, add a scant few drops of clary sage or cypress essential oils to a warm (not hot) bath a couple of hours before retiring. If the bath water is too hot, it not only has a generally enervating effect, but can also trigger a night sweat.

homeopathy

Pulsatilla This remedy is indicated for night sweats that have you hauling the bedcovers off and on in an effort to reach a stable, comfortable temperature. A stuffy bedroom may not help, but it is difficult to achieve a balance between feeling too hot and feeling too chilly.

Sulphur When getting over-heated in bed is so tormenting that you find yourself pushing both feet out of the covers to cool down, this remedy may help. In this case, the skin tends to become over-heated very quickly, but remains hot and dry rather than breaking into a sweat.

Lachesis This helps to relieve night sweats that are combined with tension, anxiety and panic. Other symptoms include an unpleasant falling sensation on drifting off to sleep that shocks you awake, followed by a sweat with palpitations and a fear of suffocating.

relaxation

If night sweats appear to be associated with a high-stress lifestyle, invest some time in learning how to switch off and relax effectively. Excellent choices to consider include meditation and visualization techniques (pages 48–49), autogenic training (pages 54–55), and progressive muscular relaxation (see Yoga, pages 56–57).

diabetes

Diabetes is the result of the body failing to produce enough insulin to regulate blood sugar levels. Type 1 (juvenile onset) diabetes can develop during childhood regardless of build and eating habits. Type 2 (adult onset) diabetes commonly occurs in people aged over 50, especially if they eat a lot of carbohydrates and refined sugar, are overweight and get little exercise. The symptoms listed below apply to both types.

common symptoms

- **Persistent thirst**
- **Frequent passing of large amounts of urine (often out of proportion to the amount of liquid taken in)**
- **Unexplained weight loss**
- **Boils and skin infections that are reluctant to heal**
- **Thrush**
- **Blurred vision**
- **Fuzzy-headedness, lack of mental focus and/or persistent tiredness**
- **Abdominal pain**
- **Nausea**

conventional treatments

If left untreated, diabetes can lead to blindness, circulatory problems such as leg ulcers, kidney failure and an increased risk of heart disease and stroke

In Type 1 diabetes, treatment involves the strict monitoring of blood sugar levels throughout the day and taking measured doses of insulin. Sugar and carbohydrate intake must also be monitored to ensure that blood sugar levels remain stable and do not fall too low (a condition known as hypoglycaemia, which can lead to coma).

In the ideal situation, Type 2 diabetes is managed by restricting the amount of refined white sugar in the diet. Regular monitoring of blood sugar levels is necessary, either by testing a drop of blood (the most accurate method) or by testing a urine sample with dip strips (less accurate). If dietary measures fail to control the situation, oral medication may be necessary to bring blood sugar levels down to a more acceptable level.

complementary treatments

Because both types of diabetes are very serious, with the potential for serious complications, both require the attention of a very experienced practitioner who is willing and able to work alongside a conventional doctor.

nutritional approaches

These will focus on eating to keep blood sugar levels as stable as possible.

other therapies to consider

If you wish to consult a trained practitioner, consider one of the following:
- Nutritional medicine
- Western medical herbalism
- Chinese herbalism
- Naturopathy

thyroid problems

Our ability to keep a range of health problems at bay depends on the healthy, balanced functioning of the thyroid gland. Some symptoms of thyroid imbalance build up insidiously (especially on reaching middle age) and can often go unnoticed until they start to interfere with quality of life. If any combination of the symptoms listed below appears after middle age and become severe, it is worth consulting your doctor.

common symptoms

Under-active thyroid

- **Constant tiredness**
- **Chilliness**
- **Unexplained weight gain**
- **Constipation**
- **Dry skin**
- **Lowered libido**

Over-active thyroid

- **Anxiety and restlessness**
- **Palpitations (fluttering heartbeat)**
- **Sleep problems**
- **A tendency to rapidly over-heat**
- **Trembling**
- **Weight loss**
- **Slightly protruding eyes**

conventional treatments

A blood test will confirm a diagnosis of under-active or over-active thyroid gland. Treatment for an under-active thyroid usually involves the use of supplements to restore a healthy level of thyroxine (the thyroid hormone). Treatment of an over-active thyroid gland involves the use of anti-thyroid drugs or surgical removal of part of the gland.

complementary treatments

Like diabetes, both conditions require the attention of a trained complementary practitioner, who will be in a position to administer appropriate treatment alongside conventional therapy. The back-up of conventional treatment is essential, because regular blood tests are necessary to establish how well the condition is being controlled. The complementary therapies listed below may be a useful addition to more conventional treatment.

therapies to consider

If you wish to consult a trained practitioner, consider one of the following:

Eastern therapies
- Chinese herbalism

Natural therapies
- Nutritional therapy
- Naturopathy
- Homoeopathy
- Western herbalism

back pain

This very common problem can have a major effect on our overall quality of life. Symptoms vary in intensity and frequency, depending on the nature of the problem. Common triggers are listed below. Back pain can either take the form of a one-off bout of acute, severe pain or it can be more of an ongoing feature of life.

common triggers

- **Muscle strain**
- **Poor postural habits**
- **A displaced disc**
- **A trapped nerve**
- **Osteoporosis**
- **Underlying illness, such as a kidney infection**

conventional treatments

Depending on the cause, treatment of back pain may involve pain-killers or anti-inflammatory drugs, steroid injections or physiotherapy. In cases of chronic back pain stemming from a mechanical problem, surgery may be necessary.

complementary treatments

For the successful treatment of back pain, these come into their own because so many of them (especially manipulative therapies) concentrate on dealing with the underlying imbalance that is triggering the problem. Possible options can include any of the following.

practicalities

• Avoid high heels, which can tip your centre of balance forward. Instead, make a point of wearing flatter shoes that support the foot. This encourages healthy alignment of the spine and hips.

• When carrying a heavy shoulder bag, swap shoulders regularly. Ring the changes by using a handbag. It also helps to keep down the weight of the contents!

• If you have used the same mattress for 8 or more years, think of changing it. Choose one that is not so soft that it sags, nor so hard that it feels like a board. If in doubt, ask your chiropractor or osteopath for advice.

• Take care when lifting heavy objects, being sure to use the muscles in your thighs rather than those in your back. Also avoid any sudden twisting movements.

• If you are concerned about the use of pain-killers, a TENS machine may be the answer. Free of any known side-effects, this machine can provide effective and fast pain relief. Once you have applied the self-adhesive pads you should feel no more than a mild, tingling sensation, rapidly followed by relief or reduction of the pain.

massage

Massage, apart from being extremely pleasurable, can be immensely helpful when combined with osteopathy or chiropractic. This is because a massage therapist can focus on loosening any tense muscles in the neck, shoulders, mid and lower back that may be contributing to back pain.

osteopathy and chiropractic

These therapies especially have an established track record in the treatment of the distress of back pain. In addition to the adjustments that they make during a session, therapists may also suggest extremely useful self-help measures.

naturopathy

If muscle tension is contributing to back pain, a soothing warm bath or shower may be helpful in temporarily calming and relieving pain.

western herbalism

Cooling gels based on glucosamine sulphate can provide temporary relief. Keep the gel in the fridge and apply it according to the directions on the tube.

alexander technique

This can be immensely helpful in teaching us how to break the negative postural habits that we have built up over the years. These habits can often be traced back to a childhood reaction to stressful stimuli. Once the problem areas have been identified, we will be able to deal with them.

arthritis

There are two basic forms of arthritis – both of which are chronic conditions and prone to periodic acute flare-ups. Osteoarthritis is often described as being due to 'wear and tear' and is associated with age. The cartilage at the end of the joints wears away and there is possible overgrowth of bone. Rheumatoid arthritis is an auto-immune condition that destroys the lining of the joints and can arise at any age.

common symptoms

- Heat, pain and swelling of the joints (usually the fingers, elbows, knees and toes in rheumatoid arthritis, and larger joints, such as the hips, or weight-bearing joints, such as the knees, in osteoarthritis)
- Stiffness and/or weakness of the affected joints
- Pain in the joints caused by tensing of the neighbouring muscles

conventional treatments

Treatment of both forms of arthritis usually involves a course of pain-killers or anti-inflammatory drugs to reduce the pain and swelling. In addition, the treatment of rheumatoid arthritis may involve steroids and/or chemotherapy-type medication. Severe cases may require surgical intervention in the form of shaving bone growth or joint replacement.

complementary treatments

These offer immense practical support for either form of arthritis. Any of the following self-help measures can be used alongside conventional treatments.

nutritional approaches

• Avoid red meat, dairy foods, alcohol, tomatoes, aubergines, potatoes, tea and coffee or any items that contain large amounts of chemical preservatives, colourings and flavourings. All these foods are thought to aggravate arthritic problems by making the entire system more acidic.

• Opt for foods and drinks that are thought to have a positive effect on the system when we have arthritic problems. These include pulses, brown rice (and rice cakes made from organic brown rice), whole grains and cereals, rye bread, sugar-free oatcakes, oily fish, free-range chicken, egg white from free-range eggs, unroasted, unsalted nuts, fresh fruit juices (except citrus fruits), coffee substitute or dandelion coffee, herb teas and plenty of still mineral or filtered tap water.

• Certain dietary supplements are thought to play an important role in preventing stiffness, discomfort and restricted movement in the joints. These include cod liver oil and vitamins A, B complex, C and E. Ginger also appears to have powerful anti-inflammatory properties and has been shown to reduce pain and swelling in 75 per cent of patients with rheumatoid and osteoarthritis.

• Remember that excess weight can put a strain on your joints so make an effort to keep it within healthy limits.

naturopathy

• Since the presence of too much toxic waste in our systems is thought to aggravate arthritic pain, guard against constipation. Every day, drink four large glasses of filtered water and ensure a high intake of dietary fibre by eating at least five portions of fruit and vegetables.

• Take a bath using Epsom salts, which have a reputation for relieving the pain and stiffness of arthritic joints and aching muscles in the short term. Follow the directions on the packet, making sure that bath water is not too hot and that you do not soak in the bath for more than 15 minutes.

• Take a supplement of glucosamine sulphate combined with chondroitin as a natural alternative to conventional anti-inflammatory drugs. A recent study, quoted by the Arthritis Research Council, suggests that this can reduce symptoms by up to 25 per cent.

yoga and tai chi

Gentle exercise is an ideal way of keeping your joints mobile and your muscles supple. Yoga and tai chi are particularly suitable.

osteoporosis

Osteoporosis (loss of bone density resulting in fragile, brittle bones) is largely without symptoms until it is well advanced, when bone fractures may occur. Because it is associated with a decline in oestrogen levels, post-menopausal women are substantially more at risk than men. Any of the symptoms listed below can suggest an underlying osteoporosis problem.

common symptoms

- **Pain or weakness in the joints of the hips, wrists and/or spine**
- **Easy or frequent fractures of the wrists or ankles**
- **Significant loss of height**
- **Muscle spasms and/or weakness of the pelvic floor muscles**
- **Restricted movement in the back and chest**

conventional treatments

Since the recent concerns about the safety of long-term hormone replacement therapy (HRT), treatment is now more likely to involve drugs that encourage bone-building cells to work more effectively and decrease the breakdown of bone.

complementary treatments

These tend to focus on preventive lifestyle measures that offer the best chance of protecting and maintaining bone density. If you think you may be at risk (for example, if you have a family history of osteoporosis), consult your doctor, who may recommend a bone-density scan.

Additional risk factors include a history of eating disorders, high alcohol and caffeine intake coupled with smoking, plus a sedentary lifestyle. Conventional medicine including oral steroids and thyroxin can also increase susceptibility to poor bone density.

nutritional approaches

• Our bones usually reach their peak density by our mid-30s so we should start eating for healthy bones as early as possible (ideally from our teens onwards). Foods to opt for include soya products, tofu, leafy green vegetables, small amounts of oily fish, fresh seeds and nuts, and small amounts of organic dairy products.

• Avoid items that have an adverse effect on bone density, such as fizzy drinks, high-protein foods, too much alcohol, caffeinated drinks, sodium-rich foods (mostly snacks, such as crisps and convenience foods that are also rich in additives) and smoked preserved meats.

naturopathy

Give up smoking if you are concerned about having healthy, strong bones. Apart from being life-threatening, smoking has been shown to accelerate signs of early ageing, such as the emergence of wrinkles, as well as reducing the production of oestrogen, which encourages calcium to leach from the bones (an effect enhanced by heavy drinking). This situation can encourage an early menopause and therefore an increased risk of osteoporosis.

exercise

Regular weight-bearing exercise plays a vital role in promoting and protecting bone density. Benefits include increased strength and stamina, as well increased oestrogen production in women. Like a healthy diet, we should start a regular exercise programme before our bones have reached maximum density for maximum benefit. Ideal types of exercise include cycling, brisk 'power-walking', low-impact aerobics, dancing, weight-training, tennis or yoga.

cramp

This unpleasant and painful problem is usually related to muscular spasms of the calf, hands or feet, although mild to excruciating cramps of the womb may also be felt during a period. It may also occur during pregnancy or vigorous exercise. The severe pain, which can last from a few seconds to several minutes, results from the sudden unexpected contraction of a muscle.

common triggers

- **Fluid loss through perspiration that also encourages the body to lose salt**
- **Fluid loss through perspiration**

common symptoms

- **Episodes of pain that can develop sharply in the affected mucle (for instance in the lower legs and feet)**
- **Slowly developing muscle cramps that build to a crescendo (as in severe period pains)**

conventional treatments

A doctor may recommend a course of quinine tablets. Alternatively, taking a small amount of salt regularly each day may resolve the problem, especially in very hot weather, when perspiring heavily may lead to loss of fluid and salt.

complementary treatments

Any of the following self-help measures can be used alongside conventional treatment.

ayurveda/ western herbalism

A warm compress of ginger can soothe the distress of a muscle cramp when gently applied to the painful area. Apart from its soothing properties, ginger also stimulates the circulation, thus easing the pain of a cramp.

Make a strong infusion of ginger, soak a soft cloth in the comfortably hot liquid before wringing it thoroughly.

aromatherapy

Massage the affected area with a cramp-banishing blend made from 3 drops each of French basil and honey myrtle to 2 teaspoonsfuls of carrier oil.

homeopathy

Arnica This remedy can be especially helpful when cramp arises from muscular over-exertion or over-engagement in unaccustomed physical activity. It is especially helpful for banishing writer's cramp, which affects the fingers.

Cuprum metallicum (Cuprum met.) Cramping pains that tend to affect the left side may be helped by this remedy. Muscles in spasm feel knotted and tremble and shake. The most commonly affected areas are the fingers, toes and calf muscles.

Nux vomica This is specific for cramps that are related to a general state of muscle tension and stress. Symptoms include a persistent desire to stretch the feet because of tightness in the calf muscles and soles of the feet. The arms may also feel periodically numb and stiff and have a tendency to 'go to sleep'.

nutritional approaches

• If cramp is a periodical problem, pay attention to your diet, ensuring that it is of a high quality so that there is a reduced risk of nutritional deficiencies or imbalances being a problem. With this aim in mind, make sure that the following are eaten on a regular basis: bananas, green leafy vegetables, whole grains, seeds, unsalted nuts and seeds, and soya products.

• In addition, specific vitamins and minerals can positively discourage cramps. These include calcium, magnesium, potassium, iron and vitamins C, D and E. If your stress levels have been high and the quality of your diet has suffered as a result, it may be worth taking a balanced multi-vitamin and multi-mineral formula. This can give you a nutritional boost as well as getting your eating patterns back on track.

naturopathy

• If a spasm of cramp affects the hand, slowly straighten and spread the fingers while pressing down gently on a firm surface.

• For foot cramps, this foot bath may help to stimulate the circulation.

Add 1 teaspoonful of powdered mustard to 2 litres (3–4 pints) of hot water and soak your tired feet for as long as feels comfortable.

exercise

If the odd bout of cramp seems to be linked to high stress levels, consider taking up a form of movement that encourages tight muscles to stretch and relax. Options include yoga, tai chi, Pilates or specific relaxation techniques that concentrate on guided visualization or progressive muscular relaxation. These should increase the blood flow to the affected areas, thereby reducing the tendency to cramps.

sports injuries

While the benefits of keeping physically fit are undeniable (enhanced stamina, muscle strength and suppleness being just a few), it is important to bear in mind that we need to exercise safely in order to reap the maximum benefits without risk of injury. Following the tips listed will help you enjoy keeping fit while reducing the possibility of problems.

hints

- **Always warm up and cool down before and after any exercise.**
- **Make sure that your shoes are designed for the purpose and fit comfortably as well as firmly supporting the foot (especially for running and particularly if this is done on a hard surface).**
- **Build up fitness levels slowly and steadily (if you have been a confirmed couch potato do not leap into a really strenuous exercise programme).**

conventional treatments

Applying an anti-inflammatory gel to the painful areas may be enough to relieve localized muscle fatigue and aching. More severe injuries may require physiotherapy or, possibly, the use of a TENS machine for pain relief.

complementary treatments

These can be invaluable in helping to speed up recovery from sports injuries and providing an extra avenue of pain relief. Any of the following measures can be used in combination with conventional medical support.

massage

Remedial massage can be incredibly helpful in relaxing tight, tense, aching muscles, especially if it is combined with chiropractic or osteopathy treatments.

osteopathy and chiropractic

These can both be immensely helpful in rectifying areas of misalignment that may be causing pain and stiffness. Practitioners of both therapies can also advise you about ways of correcting postural problems. These may be the result of carrying a heavy bag on one shoulder or wearing high-heeled shoes that affect the healthy alignment of hips and spine.

homeopathy

Arnica This is notably effective in relieving the generalized aching and stiffness that can set in after unaccustomed or prolonged or too vigorous exercise.

Rhus toxicodendron (Rhus tox.) This remedy is a specific for aching large muscles that feel incredibly uncomfortable when resting but are temporarily relieved by gentle movement or a warm bath or shower.

Bryonia This remedy is more suitable for muscle and joint pains that are considerably improved by keeping still.

naturopathy

Glucosamine sulphate is a natural, anti-inflammatory, pain-relieving gel. Pleasantly cooling when it has been stored in the fridge, apply this to stiff, sore areas as suggested in the instructions.

western herbalism

Arnica cream can soothe over-worked, aching muscles or help to speedily heal tissues that have been bruised during working out. Apply in circular movements to the affected areas, avoiding any areas of broken skin.

tendonitis

This condition commonly results from the enthusiastic playing of a particular sport (such as tennis or golf), where the tendons that attach the muscles to the bones become inflamed and painful. The most commonly affected areas are the heel and the elbow, hence the terms 'tennis elbow' and 'Achilles tendon'. This problem is more likely to develop if you exercise sporadically or neglect to warm up before exercise.

common symptoms

- **Pain and tenderness, especially on moving the affected area**
- **Restricted movement**

conventional treatments

The initial treatment is likely to involve anti-inflammatory and/or pain-relieving drugs. If these fail to resolve the problem, physiotherapy, ultrasound treatment and/or a steroid injection into the affected area may be necessary.

complementary treatments

These can be particularly useful because a complementary therapy that works well can speed up the overall healing process. Any of the following options can be considered alongside conventional medical treatment. In addition a number of other therapies are also suggested.

acupuncture

This can reduce pain while also stimulating the recovery of damaged or inflamed tissues.

osteopathy

Soft-tissue manipulation of the area can ease stiffness and limited mobility.

nutritional approaches

Certain nutrients are thought to boost the body's anti-inflammatory potential, and it is well worth taking these for conditions like tendonitis. They include fish and flaxseed oils and anti-oxidants, such as vitamins A, C and E and the trace element selenium.

therapies to consider

If you wish to consult a trained practitioner, consider one of the following:

Manipulative therapies
- Massage
- Chiropractic

Natural therapies
- Homeopathy
- Naturopathy
- Western herbalism

repetitive strain injury

Repetitive strain injury (RSI) has been increasingly recognized in recent years and appears to result from prolonged repetitive movements, so keyboard workers, assembly line workers and musicians are particularly at risk. Poorly managed stress levels, lack of breaks and/or negative postural habits appear to aggravate the problem.

common symptoms

- **Pain**
- **Weakness**
- **Tingling**

conventional treatments

Treatment usually includes advice about rest, localized support (such as a splint) and the prescription of painkillers and/or anti-inflammatory drugs. In severe cases, a doctor may suggest oral steroids to reduce inflammation.

complementary treatments

These focus on trying to find an overall solution to the problem. Any of the following self-help measures may relieve the symptoms.

practicalities

- Because poor posture may be the primary cause of RSI, it is always helpful to investigate this further. Ask an occupational health advisor at work if there are any practical measures that you can take, such as adjusting the height of your desk or chair, or using a wrist rest when working at a keyboard.

- If RSI is related to high stress levels, consider ways of relaxing more effectively, such as meditation (see pages 48–49), autogenic training (see pages 54–55) and relaxation techniques, such as progressive muscular relaxation (see page 10).

yoga

Regular yoga sessions may help people suffering from RSI. A study published in the *British Medical Journal* in 2001 showed a noticeable improvement in 42 people with carpal tunnel syndrome (which is closely associated with RSI) who had practised yoga for 8 weeks.

high blood pressure

High blood pressure can be symptomless and is often only picked up during routine medical examinations. It is a concern, however, due to its association with problems such as heart disease or stroke. A healthy blood pressure reading for women aged 30–50 is about 120/80, slightly increasing with age. Pregnancy, taking the contraceptive pill or hormone replacement therapy may affect blood pressure and call for regular monitoring.

common symptoms

- **A general feeling of being 'out of it' or vaguely unwell**
- **Headaches**
- **Palpitations**

Warning: If any of these symptoms are noticeable or frequent, you should have your blood pressure checked.

conventional treatments

The most common line of treatment involves the prescription of drugs designed to lower blood pressure (beta-blockers or angiotensin-converting enzyme (ACE) inhibitors). These may be prescribed alongside diuretic drugs aimed at encouraging the body to eliminate fluid. You may also be advised about positive lifestyle changes, such as lowering salt intake, reducing the amount of dietary fat and managing stress.

complementary treatments

Because the consequences of untreated high blood pressure can be serious, treatment is best left to an experienced practitioner. However, any of the following self-help measures may be a useful addition to any conventional or complementary treatments.

practicalities

• If you are concerned about high blood pressure, get it checked at your doctor's surgery. Blood pressure should be routinely monitored every 3 years or so, or more frequently if your doctor or practice nurse so advises.

• If you are genuinely overweight, it may help to lose a few pounds by adopting a healthy eating and exercise plan. For general suggestions on achieving and maintaining a healthy weight, see Weight gain (pages 196–97).

• Regular gentle, rhythmical exercise appears to benefit the heart and circulatory system. 'Power' walking, cycling, swimming and dancing are ideal.

• Smokers should make it a priority to kick the habit, since studies have shown that smokers with high blood pressure run an increased risk of complications.

• Drink plenty of water if you are taking diuretic drugs to control high blood pressure.

nutritional approaches

• It is important to reduce your salt intake because sodium-rich foods encourage high blood pressure. Avoid using salt at the table and in cooking, and also be aware of the 'hidden' sources in snacks, crisps, convenience foods, preserved meats such as salami and take-away meals (especially Chinese foods, which tend to contain large amounts of monosodium glutamate).

• Moderate your intake of foods containing saturated animal fats, such as red meat, full-fat cheeses, cream and lard.

• Watch your caffeine intake, because caffeine is known to increase high blood pressure, especially if you have a high-pressure lifestyle. The same applies to alcohol. To keep blood pressure within healthy limits, drink caffeine-free herb teas or coffee substitutes and have several alcohol-free nights a week.

• Opt for foods that contribute positively to the health of the heart, such as whole grains, pulses, fresh fruit and vegetables, green tea and plenty of filtered water or mineral water.

relaxation

If you have a high-stress lifestyle and struggle with high blood pressure, it will be immensely helpful to include some form of relaxation in your daily routine. Consider learning how to meditate or take up yoga or tai chi.

coronary heart disease

The coronary arteries supply the heart with oxygen and nutrients, so their health is essential. However, over time, they may become clogged up by fatty deposits (atherosclerosis) which stop them working efficiently. It is thus more likely that a clot will form, possibly causing a heart attack and eventual heart failure. Problems often come to light if the heart is required to beat faster in response to physical demands or sudden stress.

common symptoms

Atherosclerosis

- **Angina – temporary pain radiating from the heart, relieved by a short rest**
- **Breathlessness**
- **Pain in one hand and/or arm**

Heart attack

- **Pain over breast bone or left side of chest, often radiating to left arm or jaw that may last several minutes to hours**
- **Sweating and greyness of the skin**
- **Collapse**
- **Stroke**

Heart failure

- **Tiredness**
- **Breathlessness**
- **Swollen ankles**

conventional treatments

Doctors may prescribe drugs to lower blood cholesterol levels and improve blood flow in order to reduce the burden on the heart. Surgical options include angioplasty to open furred-up arteries or a coronary artery by-pass operation.

complementary medicines

These are likely to focus on improving those aspects of lifestyle known to encourage the health of the heart and circulatory system. Any of the therapies described below can be used alongside conventional treatments.

naturopathy

One of the single most positive lifestyle changes you can make is to give up smoking, since this has been shown to damage the artery walls.

nutritional approaches

Cut down drastically on the unhealthy fats in your diet. Vegetables, fruit, small amounts of cold-pressed olive oil, a glass of red wine a day and garlic are all thought to encourage a healthy heart and circulatory system.

therapies to consider

If you wish to consult a trained practitioner, consider one of the following:

Eastern therapies
- Chinese herbalism

Manipulative therapies
- Reflexology

Natural therapies
- Aromatherapy
- Homeopathy
- Naturopathy
- Western herbalism

angina

This tends to be triggered by physical exertion, emotional stress or shock. Pain occurs because the heart muscle is temporarily deprived of oxygen, normally supplied by the coronary arteries. A fit and healthy person should be able to engage in the odd burst of physical effort without feeling more than mildly out of breath. However, someone suffering from coronary heart disease may find it produces the symptoms listed below.

common symptoms

- **Pain radiating from the centre of the chest to the arms and/or neck and jaw, which clears up after rest or use of conventional medication**
- **Tight, heavy and dull pain**
- **Peripheral pains, for example in the neck, arms or wrists**
- **Dizziness, breathlessness and clamminess**

conventional treatments

Treatment consists of a spray or a tablet of nitrate drugs that can be placed under the tongue. These drugs improve the blood supply to the heart and may be suggested alongside a gentle exercise programme. Your doctor may also advise dietary changes, such as keeping your intake of saturated fats as low as possible and eating healthy portions of unrefined carbohydrates.

complementary treatments

Any of the complementary therapies listed below can provide helpful support if you have angina, but do put your doctor or cardiologist in the picture.

therapies to consider

If you wish to consult a trained practitioner, consider one of the following:

Eastern therapies
- Chinese herbalism
- Shiatsu

Manipulative therapies
- Reflexology

Natural therapies
- Homeopathy
- Nutritional therapy
- Naturopathy
- Western herbalism

Active therapies:
- Tai chi
- Yoga

chilblains

Chilblains are a mild form of frostbite and most commonly appear on the toes or fingers after exposure to the cold. They are thought to be caused by damage to the small blood vessels (capillaries) that supply the extremities of the body, which results in a reduction in the blood supply to the affected areas. The situation is not helped by a sluggish circulation.

common symptoms

- **A small white patch on an exposed part of the body, such as a finger or toe, or even the nose or ears**
- **Intense itching of the affected area, alternating with pain**
- **A red spot that develops into a small ulcer**

conventional treatments

Creams to relieve the pain and itching may be bought over the counter, or a doctor may prescribe drugs to boost the circulation. This is especially important for the elderly or people with diabetes.

complementary treatments

These tend to focus on gently improving the circulation. Any of the following self-help measures can be used in addition to conventional treatment.

practicalities

• One of the best ways of avoiding chilblains is to protect vulnerable areas, especially in bitterly cold weather. Keep your hands and feet warmly wrapped up – and do not forget your ears!

• Never be tempted to warm up freezing cold hands and feet in front of a hot fire. This is a big mistake, because it can make existing chilblains worse or even help to create them. Instead, thaw out your fingers or toes gently by immersing them in warm water.

• Bathe the affected area in warm water. Like gentle movement, this may be temporarily soothing. This is probably because both stimulate the circulation in the affected areas.

aromatherapy

Add 2 drops of lavender and tea tree essential oils to 1 teaspoonful of carrier oil and massage it gently into the problem area.
Warning Only use these oils on areas of unbroken skin.

homeopathy

Rhus toxicodrendon (Rhus tox.)
This remedy can soothe maddeningly itchy, burning chilblains that become considerably more sensitive and uncomfortable in cold, wet weather.

Petroleum This remedy is indicated for the purple-tinged chilblains that are often associated with generally dry, cracked skin that bleeds easily. These chilblains

can be incredibly painful, with a tendency for raw, burning sensations to develop.

Agaricus Chilblains that develop in areas where the skin tends to bruise readily may be eased by this remedy. The affected areas look and feel hot, swollen and red. The irritating itching changes location on scratching and touch and contact with cold air may make the discomfort worse.

nutritional approaches

Foods rich in calcium are thought to ease problems with chilblains so make a point of including them in your diet. Fresh, green leafy vegetables, almonds and small portions of organic, free-range dairy products are all excellent sources of calcium.

naturopathy

If the circulation in your hands and feet tends to be poor, gently massaging the fingers and toes each day can be helpful. This helps to stimulate the blood supply to these areas.

western herbalism

Apply Tammus cream to any areas that are cracked, painful and sensitive.
Rhus toxicodendron cream is better for distractingly itchy chilblains.

exercise

This is one of the best ways of stimulating a slightly sluggish circulation. Choose your exercise plan carefully, matching it to your overall level of starting fitness. If you have any doubts about your fitness (especially if you have a history of heart or circulatory problems), consult your doctor before starting on a fitness regime. One of the most beneficial forms of exercise that has huge benefits for the circulation is walking each day. Aim for a brisk pace (but not so much that it makes you breathless) for half an hour each day.

raynaud's syndrome

This circulatory problem is triggered by the small blood vessels that supply the fingers and toes becoming hypersensitive to cold. These contract in response to minor temperature changes but are very slow to relax again. In the early stage, warming the affected area will restore normal circulation within 15 minutes. Symptoms may be dramatic and can include any of those listed below in varying degrees of severity.

common symptoms

- **The tips of the fingers or toes turn white or greyish blue**
- **Fingers may feel tingly, burning, and/or painful**

common triggers

- **Sluggish circulation**
- **Drugs for high blood pressure**
- **Another condition, such as rheumatoid arthritis**
- **Using vibrating equipment for a long time**

conventional treatments

Apart from stressing the importance of keeping the extremities warm in cold weather, a doctor may prescribe drugs to relax and open the blood vessels.

complementary treatments

These will be aimed at generally improving the circulation of each individual. Any of the complementary treatments listed below may be helpful.

practicalities

- Wear warm gloves and socks to keep the hands and feet snug, especially during the cold winter months.

- Eat foods that are rich in vitamin E, which is thought to benefit the circulation overall. Opt for wheatgerm products and nuts, or consider taking a supplement.

Warning If you suffer from high blood pressure, ask a nutritionist for advice on a suitable dose of vitamin E.

therapies to consider

If you wish to consult a trained practitioner, consider one of the following:

Eastern therapies
- Ayurveda
- Chinese herbalism
- Shiatsu

Manipulative therapies
- Osteopathy
- Chiropractic
- Reflexology

Natural therapies
- Homeopathy
- Nutritional therapy
- Naturopathy
- Western herbalism

thread veins

These areas of tiny, purplish veins on the surface of the skin often appear on the upper and lower legs, or where the skin is quite thin. They result from blockages in the tiny blood vessels (capillaries) or damage to their walls.

common triggers

- **Hereditary factors**
- **Hormonal changes (for instance approaching or following menopause)**
- **Injury**
- **Steroid creams**

conventional treatments

These are mainly cosmetic and involve the use of a very mild electric current to stem the flow of blood to the damaged capillary, thus making the thread vein less visible. Alternatively, a blockage can be removed by injecting a special solution.

complementary treatments

As with all circulatory problems, any complementary approach will focus on ways of improving the functioning of the circulatory system. Suitable therapies are listed below. In addition, some of the practical measures listed may help.

practicalities

- Avoid very hot water for bathing the face or areas of thinner skin, or where thread veins are already visible, as this can further damage the capillary walls.

- Breathing techniques, especially with exercise, can help to tone the circulatory system. Breathe in slowly and deeply, filling as much of your lungs as possible. Breathe out slowly to expel the carbon dioxide as efficiently as possible.

nutritional approaches

Certain foods may be beneficial, such as apricots, citrus fruit, grapes, blackberries, cherries, broccoli, avocados, buckwheat, wheatgerm, and nuts and seeds.

therapies to consider

If you wish to consult a trained practitioner, consider one of the following:

Eastern therapies
- Ayurveda

Natural therapies
- Homeopathy
- Nutritional therapy
- Naturopathy
- Western herbalism

varicose veins

These result from too much blood seeping into the superficial veins of the legs. This happens when the valves that should prevent the back-flow of blood into the veins become weak. They most commonly affect the thigh, calf, groin or ankle. Varicose veins often develop during or after pregnancy, if our job involves a lot of standing or after middle age. Symptoms, which vary in severity, are listed below.

common symptoms

- Throbbing, aching or itching of the skin surrounding or covering the distended vein
- A knobbly, bluish appearance to the swollen veins, especially after standing
- Discomfort that is more noticeable in the days before or during a period
- Varicose ulcers – caused by the breakdown of the skin over a varicose vein

conventional treatments

For mild problems, this usually involves practical advice about taking regular exercise, such as walking, and using support tights when standing for long periods. More severe or well-established problems may require surgery.

complementary treatments

Any of the following can be used alongside conventional treatment in order to ease mild to moderate problems with varicose veins.

practicalities

• Rest with your feet slightly raised so that the blood in the veins of the legs drains more effectively and the veins appear less swollen.

• Wear support tights or stockings to support aching varicose veins and give temporary relief from aching and discomfort. You should avoid hold-up stockings, however, since the tight elastic at the top of the thigh can aggravate problems with varicose veins.

• Regular exercise, such as brisk walking, conditions and protects the circulatory system, since the contraction and relaxation of the muscles in the legs propels the blood through the veins. Standing has the reverse effect, encouraging the blood to pool in the veins.

aromatherapy

Seek the advice of a qualified practitioner, who will be able to make up a blend tailored for your situation. Use this as directed by the practitioner.

homeopathy

Hamamelis This is one of the most commonly used homeopathic treatments for general symptoms of painful, swollen varicose veins. Sensations are bruising of a prickling nature, coupled with a tendency to develop chilblains.

Arnica Use this remedy to soothe to varicose veins that are excruciatingly sensitive to the touch. Pains may be combined with marked restlessness and a tendency to constantly move the feet in an effort to ease the bruised, aching sensations in the legs.

nutritional approaches

Eat more of the foods that have a reputation for strengthening blood vessels, stimulating a sluggish circulation and encouraging the draining of excess fluid from the tissues. These include grapes, citrus fruit, spinach, parsley, buckwheat, garlic, green cabbage and dandelion.

naturopathy

Avoid standing in one position for longer than necessary and try not to sit cross-legged since this can put additional pressure on the veins of the legs.

western herbalism

A compress of Calendula infusion can ease the pain and swelling of sore veins.

Dilute 1 part Calendula tincture to 10 parts cooled, boiled water. Soak a length of clean, soft gauze in it, wring out the excess liquid and apply the gauze to the sore, aching area.

swollen glands

We tend to become aware of our glands only when they become painful or swollen – a sign that our immune systems are fighting infection. The areas most commonly affected are the neck, armpits and groin, and the symptoms should subside once the infection is over. However, any low-level swelling of the glands, which either remains or comes and goes, requires medical advice.

common causes

- **Fighting an acute infection if the glands come up speedily and go down once the infection is over**
- **Illnesses that involve glandular swelling and tenderness, including tonsilitis, flu, glandular fever and mumps**

conventional treatments

A short episode of swollen glands may resolve itself, in which case, treatment may not be necessary. If you have a more severe or established problem, your doctor may arrange some tests, such as a blood test for glandular fever.

Other chronic problems that can lead to persistent or intermittent swollen glands may be related to chronic fatigue syndrome, lymphoma or Hodgkin's disease.

complementary treatments

A course of complementary or alternative therapy may considerably benefit intermittent episodes of benign swollen glands. The treatments below aim to support the body in resolving one-off episodes of minor glandular swelling.

Should low-grade swelling appear to be linked to the body's inability to fight infection efficiently (this would need to be confirmed by your family doctor), this is a situation where you should consider seeking professional complementary medical help.

homeopathy

Bryonia This can ease the acute pain of glandular swelling that is made worse by even the slightest movement. Symptoms tend to develop slowly and insidiously over a few days, often after exposure to dry, cold winds.

Mercurius Swollen glands accompanied by a sore throat, with bad breath and a metallic taste in the mouth may be soothed by this remedy.
Warning It is best not to use Mercurius if you have a high fever.

Pulsatilla Swollen glands that linger at the end of a nasty cold. The mouth may feel dry and the tongue look like it is coated with white 'fur'. Glandular swelling may be worse or confined to the right side of the body.

Hepar sulphuris calcareum (Hepar sulph.) This remedy helps reduce the discomfort of swollen glands that are associated with a nasty sore throat or ear infection. Mucus is likely to be nasty, thick and yellowy-green in colour.

naturopathy

If salivary glands are painful it helps to avoid any food or drinks that are tart or acidic in flavour. These have the unfortunate effect of stimulating salivary activity which can feel very uncomfortable.

therapies to consider

If you wish to consult a trained practitioner, consider one of the following:

- Naturopathy

- Homeopathy

- Western herbalism

- Chinese herbalism

post-viral syndrome

This debilitating condition (also known as chronic fatigue syndrome or myalgic encephalomyelitis, ME) often affects high achievers, who tend to push themselves too hard. Dealing with it may be a problem, since controversy still exists in conventional medical circles about whether or not it is a medical condition. This is due partly to the lack of any definitive diagnostic test and partly to the extremely variable symptoms.

common symptoms

- **Extreme physical, mental and emotional exhaustion**
- **Aching muscles**
- **Digestive problems**
- **Sleep disturbance**
- **Recurrent infections**
- **Glandular swelling**
- **Anxiety and depression**
- **Headaches**

conventional treatments

There is no definitive treatment for this condition but avenues of support include the prescription of antidepressants, counselling or stress management advice. If recurrent infections are a problem, a doctor may suggest antibiotics or anti-fungal preparations.

complementary treatments

These treatments are extremely well placed to give broad-based, medical support for post-viral syndrome. For the best results, you should consult an experienced practitioner. In addition, any of the following self-help measures can be useful.

naturopathy

• Regular dry skin-brushing can encourage the body to detoxify. Use a natural bristle brush on dry skin, moving over your body in firm but gentle upward strokes before bathing or showering.

• In addition, drink six to eight large glasses of still mineral water or filtered tap water every day to help the body eliminate toxic waste.

nutritional approaches

• If yeast infections are a persistent problem, it may help to eat garlic and natural bio-yoghurt every day. Supplements of caprylic acid or acidophilus can support the body in dealing with persistent candida overgrowth.

• Since post-viral syndrome develops when the immune system is overloaded and struggling to fight infection, it is sensible to adopt eating patterns that support the body's defences. Avoid junk foods, which contain large amounts of synthetic flavourings, colourings and preservatives, and any items (such as alcohol, sugar and large amounts of protein) that put an extra strain on the organs of detoxification – the kidneys and the liver.

• As well as eating fresh, natural foods (wholegrains, pulses, small amounts of fish, and raw fruit and vegetables), it may help to take supplements that support the functioning of the immune system. These include the anti-oxidant vitamins A, C and E, plus the trace elements selenium and zinc.

• The herbal remedy Echinacea may also be beneficial, but do bear mind that this should be taken in short courses rather than be adopted as a long-term strategy.

exercise

Although regular exercise has been repeatedly shown to benefit the health of body and mind, this may not be altogether true in the case of post-viral syndrome. Although a graduated regime of gentle exercise such as Pilates or yoga, can help to build-up energy levels, and benefit the system as a whole, doing too much too soon can have an energy-depleting rather than an energy-boosting effect, making the condition temporarily worse.

therapies to consider

If you wish to consult a trained practitioner, consider one of the following:

Eastern therapies
• Chinese herbalism

Manipulative therapies
• Chiropractic

Natural therapies
• Aromatherapy

• Homeopathy

• Nutritional therapy

• Naturopathy

• Western herbalism

auto immune disorders

These chronic disorders arise as a result of the body's natural defence mechanism (the immune system) turning on itself and attacking the body's own tissues. The common symptoms of all these conditions include inflammation and pain resulting from the immune system's inability to differentiate between the cells of a hostile invader and the normal cells of the body.

auto immune diseases

Examples include:

- **Rheumatoid arthritis**
- **Corneal ulcers**
- **Multiple sclerosis**

conventional treatments

These usually focus on reducing pain and inflammation as effectively as possible. Depending on the condition, treatment options include steroids and/or anti-inflammatory drugs. Because there is no clear understanding of why the immune system reacts in such an inbalanced way, effort is aimed mainly at managing the symptoms rather than finding a cure.

psychotherapy and counselling

Being told that you have an auto-immune problem, such as multiple sclerosis or rheumatoid arthritis, can be very difficult to cope with. Therefore, the chance to explore and talk through the issues with a sympathetic, objective listener can be a great help. This is especially the case when family members, a partner or friends are too emotionally involved to put things in context.

complementary treatments

Because these disorders are chronic rather than acute, they are best treated by a trained practitioner who will aim to discourage the immune system from acting in this fashion. As a result, patients should find that acute flare-ups happen less frequently, even if the underlying tendency to the problem remains. In addition, the following self-help measures may be useful.

massage

Always pleasurable and relaxing, massage can play an important supportive role in balancing immune system function. Where chronic pain is a problem, it can relax the muscles and provide the comfort of touch. This can be especially important to anyone who feels stressed, anxious and isolated as a result of the condition.

nutritional therapy

• For any condition involving the irregular functioning of the immune system, you should avoid foods and drinks that are known to place a strain on the body's defences. These include alcohol, refined sugar and a high or regular intake of hydrogenated fats.

• Instead, focus on foods that support the immune system, particularly items that are rich in anti-oxidants, such as bright red, orange and dark green vegetables.

western herbalism

Although Echinacea is thought to aid immune system functioning (for example, when fighting off an acute infection like a heavy cold), it is best not to self-prescribe in situations involving auto immune problems. Always consult an experienced practitioner of herbal medicine who will be able to decide on the support most appropriate to the circumstances.

relaxation techniques

The newly emerging science of psycho-neuro-immunology offers a fascinating perspective on the role of the mind in regularizing immune system functioning. Early studies show that regular relaxation, especially when combined with positive affirmations backed up by positive experiences, can play a significantly positive role in supporting the healthy functioning of the immune system.

therapies to consider

If you wish to consult a trained practitioner, consider one of the following:

• Homeopathy

• Chinese herbalism

• Naturopathy

• Nutritional therapy

allergic rashes

These can take the form of urticaria (nettle rash or hives) or prickly heat. Urticaria tends to be triggered by contact with or eating a substance to which you are allergic (an allergen). Prickly heat is often triggered by exposure to excessive heat and sunlight. Symptoms usually develop very quickly.

common allergens

- **Fish**
- **Nuts (especially peanuts)**
- **Strawberries**
- **Conventional drugs, such as aspirin or codeine**

common symptoms

- **Itchy, red weals that can migrate to any part of the body**
- **Rashes may be large and blotchy, or more like a series of pin-pricks**
- **Rashes may last from just a few minutes to several days**
- **There may no obvious pattern or trigger, with outbreaks being randomly intermittent**

Warning: If symptoms are severe, with signs of swelling around the lips and/or throat, you should seek urgent emergency treatment.

conventional treatments

These focus on reducing the inflammation and irritation as quickly as possible and usually involve the prescription of antihistamines or, in more severe cases, steroids.

complementary treatments

Since the existence of a chronic skin condition is always the sign of a deeper underlying disorder, you should always consult a skilled practitioner. In addition, any of the following self-help measures can temporarily relieve the irritation and itching.

aromatherapy

Add 4 or 5 drops of chamomile or melissa essential oils to a warm (not hot) bath to soothe the irritation. If the bath water is too hot, it can aggravate the sensitivity and irritation of the skin.

homeopathy

Apis This can ease the irritation and stinging of large, raised, rosy pink hives. The affected areas may appear to be waterlogged and are painfully sensitive to heat in any form.

Arsenicum album Small, pin-prick rashes that are temporarily eased and soothed by contact with warmth (such as a warm compress or warm bath) are more suited to this remedy. When at their most sensitive, the spots burn violently.

Rhus toxicodendron (Rhus tox.) This can temporarily soothe small, blistery, fluid-filled hives that are particularly bothersome at night. They can develop after getting chilled and wet, and the skin feels much worse for contact with cold draughts of air.

Hepar sulphuris calcareum (Hepar sulph.) For temporary relief from the itching and distress of well-established skin allergies, where the skin becomes easily infected, try this remedy. Because the skin is hypersensitive, there may also be considerable mental irritability and over-sensitivity.

western herbalism

If the skin is stinging and burning as well as itchy, the following may give temporary relief.

Add 1 part of Urtica urens tincture to 10 parts of cooled water and, using a cottonwool pad, dab on the affected area as often as necessary.

bach flower remedies

Apply Rescue Remedy cream to the hot, itchy, irritated skin as often as necessary.

therapies to consider

If you wish to consult a trained practitioner, consider one of the following:

Eastern therapies
• Ayurveda
• Chinese herbalism

Natural therapies
• Homeopathy
• Nutritional therapy
• Naturopathy
• Western herbalism

allergic rhinitis

Allergic rhinitis is rather like having hay fever all year round. Basically, it is an over-reaction of the eyes, nose, throat and/or chest to contact with an airborne substance. This releases histamine which triggers the inflammation and streaming of the eyes and nose. Symptoms vary greatly in their frequency, severity and duration. You may notice that symptoms are predictably worse on first waking or in the morning.

common symptoms

- **Bloodshot eyes which feel gritty and sensitive**
- **Watery eyes that stream continually**
- **Irritation of the eyes and eyelids**
- **Streaming and/or obstruction of the nose**
- **Constant sneezing**
- **Itchy, dry throat**
- **Wheezing**

conventional treatments

These focus on reducing inflammation, irritation and congestion in the nose, eyes and chest, and usually involves the prescription of steroid eye or nasal drops, as well as inhalers. Antihistamines, to reduce the symptoms of allergic response, are another treatment option.

complementary treatments

These aim to deal with the underlying imbalance in the system that is causing the symptoms to emerge, and they may take some time to have an effect. In addition, any of the following self-help measures may substantially relieve the acute symptoms in the short-term. Complementary treatment is generally aimed at discouraging the over-sensitivity and over-reactivity that give rise to symptoms.

practicalities

• Wherever possible, limit your exposure to substances known to aggravate allergic rhinitis. Common culprits include house-dust mites, animal fur, perfumes and fungal spores from mould and damp.

• Invest in special allergen-free covers for your mattress and pillows and avoid duvets or pillows that are filled with duck down. Scrupulous vacuuming can also pay dividends.

• Try to resist the temptation to rub your eyes because this will only encourage histamine production, which will make the swelling of the eyelids worse. Instead, bathe your eyes in cool water to relieve the irritation.

aromatherapy

For the short-term relief of nasal congestion, inhale a few drops of essential oil of peppermint from a tissue, making sure that the oil doesn't make contact with your skin.

homeopathy

Apis Puffiness around the eyes that looks pale pink and water-logged may be relieved by this remedy. The eyes may sting and water, and be very sensitive to bright light and warmth.

Allium cepa This is suitable for symptoms specifically affecting the nose, which streams so much that it makes the top lip burn. The eyes also water a lot, but the tears are bland in comparison.

Euphrasia This remedy is more suitable for symptoms that make the eyes especially uncomfortable. The eyes may feel as is they are brimming with burning tears, while the eyelids look sore, red and inflamed. Although the nose runs a lot, the discharge is relatively bland.

nutritional approaches

To help support the self-regulating mechanism of the body, avoid foods that contain chemical additives. You can also take certain supplements to help balance the immune system, such as vitamin C with bioflavonoids, vitamins of the B complex and vitamin E.

western herbalism

To help soothe itchy, sore, prickly eyes, bathe them with diluted Euphrasia tincture. Alternatively, saturate two cottonwool pads in a dilution of 1 part Euphrasia tincture to 10 parts boiled, cooled water and place them over your eyes.

food sensitivities

Food sensitivities or intolerances are particularly controversial because conventional medical opinion is divided about whether they do in fact exist or are just 'in the mind'. Unlike food allergies, they do not produce an antibody reaction in a blood test and therefore cannot be specifically identified. However, if you genuinely do have a sensitivity to wheat for instance, dramatic results can come from taking positive action.

common symptoms

- **Migraines**
- **Headaches**
- **Mood swings, including depression and anxiety**
- **Mouth ulcers**
- **Digestive problems**
- **Muscle aches and pains**
- **Poor quality skin**
- **Low energy levels**

conventional treatments

Many conventional doctors find it difficult to take on board the idea of food sensitivity, partly due to the absence of any definitive diagnostic test. As a result, there is, as yet, no established conventional treatment.

complementary treatments

Complementary treatments have far more to offer because they regard each patient as an individual and are less concerned with establishing the existence of a condition. The treatment of food sensitivities requires the expertise of a qualified medical practitioner. Nevertheless, although you should not rely on self-help measures alone, some of the following may be useful additions to treatment.

nutritional approaches

• It has been estimated that anyone eating an average Western diet, with a large proportion of foods and drinks that are high in calories but low in nutrients, may be ingesting more than 100 artificial additives each day. It is possible to have a food intolerance test, the most reliable being analysis of a blood sample.

• Once the offending item has been eliminated from the diet, it may help to take supplements that support the immune system (such as vitamins A, C and E), plus lactobacillus supplements and live bio-yoghurt to rebalance the gut flora. This can be especially helpful where food sensitivities have been triggered or made worse by a course of antibiotics.

naturopathy

The most likely course of action is an elimination diet in which any suspect food (most commonly dairy products and foods containing white sugar and/or wheat) is cut out of the diet for about 2 weeks. If this results in a marked improvement, the suspect food is re-introduced to see whether any adverse reaction occurs. This process is repeated and a second adverse reaction will suggest that there is a genuine problem. The food in question should then be avoided wherever possible, while complementary medical treatment is sought in order to strengthen and re-balance the system.

relaxation techniques

Since some of the problems associated with food sensitivities may be aggravated by high stress levels, ways of effectively switching off can be a helpful supportive measure. Options to choose from include progressive muscular relaxation, visualization techniques, autogenic training or diaphragmatic breathing.

therapies to consider

If you wish to consult a trained practitioner, consider one of the following:

Natural therapies

• Homeopathy

• Nutritional therapy

• Naturopathy

• Western herbalism

bruises

Bruises result from bleeding under the skin and the accumulation of fluid in the tissues. Depending on the nature of the injury or trauma, they can vary hugely in severity and seriousness. When bruises occur as the result of minor injury, there is seldom any cause for alarm, since the traumatized tissue will heal perfectly well in time. However, after a major accident, bruising may be a sign of serious injury.

common causes

- **Falls**
- **Heavy blows**
- **Surgery**
- **Childbirth**

common symptoms

- **Purple discoloration of the skin, fading to yellow**
- **Swelling**
- **Tenderness**

warning symptoms

Seek urgent medical attention if any of the following develop after an accident.

- **Drowsiness, nausea and/or slurred speech, especially after a severe fall or head injury**
- **Dizziness after an accident**
- **Injury to the eye**
- **Suspected internal bruising**
- **Bruises that are slow to heal, or that occur very easily and frequently**

conventional treatments

For mild bruising related to minor injury, hold a cold compress against the bruised area to relieve tenderness and swelling (provided that the surface of the skin is unbroken).

complementary treatments

These can encourage speedy healing of bruises by stimulating the efficient re-absorption of blood from the damaged tissues. Any of the following self-help measures can help to heal a minor bruise in double-quick time.

aromatherapy

Dilute essential oils of lavender or marjoram in water and apply this to bruised tissue in the form of a cool compress. This will soothe tenderness and stimulate speedy healing.

homeopathy

Arnica This is the first remedy to consider for bruising that has resulted from an accident. It not only promotes speedy resolution of the bruise by encouraging re-absorption of blood but also helps deal with the psychological shock and trauma that can accompany even the most minor accident.

Bellis perennis Next to Arnica, this does well in treating bruises that have been sustained to very deep tissue, such as a heavy blow to the breasts. It can also be incredibly helpful in resolving deep bruising that follows surgery.

Ledum This is specifically helpful for bruises that feel superficially numb and cold and are soothed by cool bathing or applying a cool compress. It is particularly suitable for black eyes, where the bruised tissue is incredibly sensitive and swollen.

Symphytum This can be immensely helpful in resolving bruising and tenderness in areas where the skin is thin (such as damage to the bony socket of the eye from a blunt object). It is also indicated where Arnica has helped initially with pain and tenderness, but failed to fully resolve the situation.

western herbalism

• Apply Arnica to the bruised area in the form of a diluted tincture, cream or massage balm to soothe and cool the pain and tenderness.
Warning Do not use Arnica on broken skin because it can trigger inflammation.

• Apply diluted witch hazel to soothe and cool tender, bruised skin.
Warning Take care if you have sensitive skin because witch hazel is highly astringent.

bach flower remedies

Apply Rescue Remedy cream to the bruise. This can be extremely helpful in soothing the surface pain and healing traumatized tissues.

bites

Bites are most commonly due to insects, such as fleas, midges, mosquitoes, and unless we are particularly sensitive, or the bite becomes infected, they cause little more than temporary intense irritation. Cat or dog bites are more serious, because of the risk of blood poisoning, and so are bites from venomous animals.

common symptoms

- **Redness, heat and inflammation**
- **Swelling and puffiness of the skin**

warning symptoms

The following symptoms suggest a major allergic reaction that needs extremely urgent medical attention.

- **Drowsiness**
- **Difficulty in breathing or rapid breathing**
- **Swelling of the face, lips and/or throat**

In addition, more serious bites (for example from a dog or a venomous animal) require prompt medical attention.

conventional treatments

For minor insect bites, cool bathing and the passage of time may suffice. It may also be wise to use an insect repellent in future (especially when on holiday).

complementary treatments

Treatments for minor bites include the following:

aromatherapy

Apply a drop of lavender oil to the affected area every hour until the irritation and discomfort stops.

homeopathy

Staphysagria This soothes the irritation of midge bites, which can be exquisitely sensitive. It can also be taken to discourage midges from biting.

western herbalism

- To relieve the irritation of stinging, itchy bites, bathe with diluted Urtica urens (1 part tincture to 10 parts cooled, boiled water). Dab on the solution as often as necessary using a cottonwool pad.

- If midge bites are likely to be a problem (especially on holiday), apply diluted feverfew tincture to the skin as a natural insect repellant. A solution of vinegar and water will achieve a similar effect (if you can cope with the smell!).

stings

The most likely stings are from wasps or bees during the summer months. Although not usually serious in themselves, the localized pain and swelling of a sting can be extremely unpleasant. However, they can be life-threatening to people who are allergic to them.

common symptoms

• Localized swelling

• Pain

• Inflammation

warning symptoms

The following symptoms suggest a major allergic reaction that needs extremely urgent medical attention.

• Drowsiness

• Difficulty in breathing or rapid breathing

• Swelling of the face, lips and/or the throat

conventional treatments

For minor reactions to a sting, which subside over time, the complementary advice below should speed up the healing process. People who know they are allergic to bee or wasp stings should consult their doctor with a view to carrying the appropriate medication with them at all times.

complementary treatments

Any of the following can help soothe the localized pain and distress of a sting.

practicalities

• In the case of a bee sting, first remove the sting with a clean pair of tweezers. Then bathe the affected area with a solution of bicarbonate of soda and water. This will to help reduce the level of pain and swelling.

• For wasp stings, apply a solution of vinegar and water. The venom in the sting is alkaline so this acidic mixture will neutralize it.

aromatherapy

Apply a drop of lavender essential oil to the sting at hourly intervals to reduce pain and inflammation.

western herbalism

• Remove the sting, check that the wound is clean and bathe it with a solution of Hypericum and Calendula tincture (1 part tincture to 10 parts cooled, boiled water). After bathing, apply Hypericum and Calendula cream. This has the dual function of easing pain and having natural antiseptic properties.

• To relieve the pain and irritation of nettle stings, gently rub a dock leaf over the affected area. However, only do this for a short time so that the skin does not become sensitized.

burns

Minor burns and scalds tend to be an everyday hazard of working in the kitchen where there are ready sources of heat in the form of kettles, ovens, hobs and irons. More serious burns will need medical attention. Take preventative action by observing safety rules, such as turning handles of saucepans away from the edge of the cooker, taking care when pouring hot liquids and keeping hot water at a sensible temperature.

common causes

- Fire
- Contact with a badly adjusted central heating radiator
- Putting the hands under a tap that dispenses extremely hot water
- Contact with corrosive cleaning chemicals

warning symptoms

Seek urgent medical attention if any of the following are present:

- Burns or scalds that cover an area greater than 2.5 cm (1 in) in diameter.
- Severe blistering
- Charred skin
- Chemical or electrical burns

conventional treatments

Hold a minor burn or scald under the cold tap until the pain eases. Then apply a soothing antiseptic cream and a dressing.

complementary treatments

Any of the following are excellent supportive measures that can help speed up the healing process of a minor burn or scald.

Complementary measures are especially helpful for the treatment of very minor burns and scalds since they can substantially speed up the natural healing process.

aromatherapy

Dilute 10 drops of lavender essential oil in a carrier oil or gel base and apply very gently to the inflamed, painful area.

homeopathy

Urtica urens This can be taken internally for minor burns that are red and burning, with a small degree of blister formation and a marked sensitivity and aversion to touch.

Arnica This can help ease general symptoms of shock that can accompany even the most minor of burns. It can be given before moving on to Urtica urens to resolve the healing process.

naturopathy

For very minor burns, apply Vitamin E oil to encourage speedy healing and discourage scarring. If you do not have a bottle of oil handy, but you do have Vitamin E oil capsules, puncture the casing with a clean pin or needle and squeeze out the oil.

western herbalism

• Apply a solution of Urtica urens tincture (1 part tincture to 10 parts cooled, boiled water) to soothe the initial pain, stinging and inflammation of a minor burn or scald. Either bathe the affected area in the solution or use a cottonwool pad to dab it on the affected area.

• If a blister has formed and been accidentally broken, use a solution of Calendula tincture (1 part tincture to 10 parts cooled, boiled water), which has naturally antiseptic properties. Follow this up by applying Calendula cream gently to the area.

• For extra pain relief combined with natural antiseptic properties, apply a combined Hypericum and Calendula cream and tincture. Hypericum helps to temporarily soothe pain in areas that are rich in nerve endings.

bach flower remedies

Dilute a few drops of Rescue Remedy in a small glass of water and sip it at regular intervals in order to alleviate any shock from a minor burn or scald.

wounds

Wounds vary hugely in size and severity, from minor grazes to deep incisions, depending on the nature of the accident that produced them. Obviously, in this book it is only appropriate to consider self-help measures for minor wounds.

warning symptoms

All major wounds require urgent medical attention.

- **Severe bleeding that cannot be stopped**
- **A wide cut that cannot be held together with standard dressings**
- **Long, jagged wounds, especially over a joint such as the knee or elbow**
- **Deeply embedded dirt that cannot be dislodged by gentle bathing**
- **Cuts to the palm of the hand or sides of the fingers**
- **Any signs of infection in or around a wound, such as redness, heat or pus, or raised temperature**

conventional treatments

For minor wounds, bathe the affected area to make sure that it is clean, apply an antiseptic cream and cover with a sterile dressing. If the edges of the wound will not to come together, stitches may be necessary.

complementary treatments

Any of the following measures can gently encourage the speedy healing of minor wounds.

homeopathy

Arnica This is the first remedy to reach for after any minor accident, trauma or injury. It not only helps to resolve bruising swiftly and efficiently, but also encourages wounds to heal. Equally importantly, it eases the psychological shock that so often accompanies even the most minor of accidents.

Warning Do not use Arnica on broken skin because it can trigger inflammation around the edge of wounds.

Hypericum This is immensely helpful in healing cuts that are near a rich nerve supply, once the situation has been checked by a doctor. It can also be very helpful in encouraging the healing of deep cuts that are extremely sensitive to touch, as well as in resolving any pain that lingers after an epidural.

Ledum Use this remedy to encourage puncture wounds to heal once they have received appropriate medical attention and when the wound is soothed by cool bathing or contact with cool compresses, or when the wound itself feels cold.

Staphysagria This is especially suitable for healing incised wounds, especially those associated with surgery or childbirth, where stitches were needed. Wounds that need this remedy are likely to sting and feel hypersensitive to touch. Staphysagria can be especially helpful after childbirth, especially if it involved an episiotomy or Caesarian. In this context, it can also help relieve some of the discomfort of catheterization.

western herbalism

• Bathe minor wounds and clean cuts in a solution of Calendula tincture (1 teaspoonful of the tincture to a small glass of cooled, boiled water). This has an all-round beneficial action, encouraging healing of tissue, acting as a natural antiseptic and helping to stop minor bleeding. Make sure that any debris has been washed out of the wound before applying Calendula cream or ointment, otherwise, the skin may heal over it, leaving infection to fester at a deeper level.

• Grazed, roughened skin may respond better to bathing in a solution of Hypericum and Calendula tincture followed by an application of the matching cream and covering with a sterile dressing.

shock

The term 'shock' can be used in several different contexts, which may lead to some confusion as to its meaning. It can refer to our response to a minor accident or distressing news, or it can refer to a life-threatening medical condition. This section refers to the former. If you suspect that a more serious shock state may be developing, lose no time in getting emergency medical help.

common symptoms

- **Dizziness**
- **Nausea**
- **Rapid heartbeat or palpitations**
- **Sweating**
- **Shaking or trembling**

warning symptoms

Seek urgent medical attention if any of the following symptoms develop.

- **Severe dizziness, leading to unconsciousness**
- **Pallor with any sign of a blue tinge around the lips or extremities**
- **Pains in the abdomen accompanied by vomiting and/or diarrhoea**
- **Noticeable swelling around the eyes, face, lips or throat**
- **Laboured and/or wheezy breathing patterns**

conventional treatments

For minor shock, sitting down with a cup of sweet tea may be sufficient to relieve the symptoms.

complementary treatments

Any of the following measures will help to bring about rapid recovery following mild shock.

homeopathy

Aconite This is very helpful in easing the panic and fear often associated with physical or emotional shock.

Arnica This remedy helps to dispel the shock reaction that is so often part-and-parcel of even the most minor of accidents. Even if there was no time to give it at the time of the incident, it can still be of value some time later.

Ignatia This can be immensely helpful as a homeopathic remedy in easing the shock and distress of bereavement. It can also be helpful to anyone who feels they are 'stuck' in a grief state and can't move on, no matter how hard they try (see also pages 86–87).

bach flower remedies

A few drops of Rescue Remedy placed directly on the tongue, or diluted in a small glass of water and sipped at regular intervals, will help calm the system and clear the mind.

fainting

A temporary loss of consciousness due to a shortage in the blood supply to the brain, this is most often caused by a drop in blood pressure or standing up too quickly. It can also be caused by shock, severe pain (for example severe period pain) or over-tiredness. Some women are more prone to fainting during pregnancy or at menopause, which may be due to fluctuating hormone levels, unstable blood sugar levels or anaemia.

common symptoms

- **Pallor**
- **Sweating**
- **Slow pulse**
- **A craving for cool air on the face**

warning symptoms

Seek urgent medical attention if any of the following symptoms develop.

- **Continuing unconsciousness**
- **Breathing problems**

conventional treatments

The standard treatment for a faint is to restore the blood supply to the brain by getting the patient to lie down with their legs slightly elevated. If he or she is over-heated, loosen any tight, restrictive clothing around the neck and waist, and check that there is nothing in the mouth that could cause choking.

complementary treatments

Any of the following can help speed up recovery and dispel shock after a minor, uncomplicated faint. If a tendency to frequent fainting is becoming a pattern, the patient could consider consulting an experienced complementary medical practitioner for advice and treatment on how to prevent the problem.

homeopathy

Carbo vegetabilis (Carbo veg.) This is the first remedy to think of when a faint has occurred.

Pulsatilla This remedy can speed recovery where fainting has occurred in response to getting over-heated in a stuffy, badly ventilated room, especially during a period or at menopause.

naturopathy

- An alternative restorative drink to the traditional cup of strong, sweet tea can be made by dissolving a dessertspoonful of honey and a pinch of cinnamon in a cup of hot water.

- If fainting is known to have been triggered by going too long without eating so that blood sugar levels have dropped sharply, a mixture of lemon juice and honey can help to ease disorientation and tiredness.

sprains

Sprains occur when the ligaments that support the ankle, knee, wrist or fingers are damaged, usually as the result of injury. They are most commonly caused by putting too much stress on the affected joint, usually as a result of a sharply jarring movement (such as turning over on an ankle) or by a fall. The degree of pain experienced relates to the amount of damage sustained by the ligaments in question.

common symptoms

- **Noticeable visible swelling of the damaged joint**
- **Discolouration and distortion of the sprained joint**

conventional treatments

Depending on the severity of the sprain, strapping the affected joint should prevent further damage to the injured ligaments. Pain-killers may be necessary to dull the pain, which can be considerable if the sprain is severe.

complementary treatments

Any of the following can be used to speed up the healing process in a mild to moderate sprain.

homeopathy

Arnica This is the first remedy to reach for after a sprain. It will reduce the initial swelling and help to relieve the pain.

Rhus toxicodendron (Rhus tox.) Next to Arnica, this remedy is ideal for the treatment of sprains where the pains are obviously worse for too much rest and are generally relieved by gentle movement that does not over-tax the joint. Warm bathing also feels very soothing, while becoming chilled or cold makes the pain more acute.

naturopathy

If the skin is intact, apply an ice pack to the affected area to reduce the swelling and reduce some of the pain temporarily. A bag of frozen peas wrapped in a soft cloth is an excellent substitute for an ice pack.

strains

These usually result from the muscles becoming over-stretched, most commonly after over-strenuous exercise or failure to warm up properly beforehand. This is due to the way that used muscle can't stretch as easily and effectively. Once the muscle fibres are damaged, the area can become swollen as the affected muscle becomes inflamed and engorged by internal bleeding.

common symptoms

- Minor muscles strains can be treated at home rather than requiring surgical intervention
- Swelling, stiffness and pain when the muscle is used

warning symptoms

- If a muscle looks as though it has been ruptured (thankfully this is a compartively rare occurrence), help is promptly needed
- If the affected muscle is excrutiatingly painful and swollen, and refuses to respond to self-help, seek a medical opinion.

conventional treatments

First rest the injured limb, then bandage it firmly enough to give support without restricting the blood flow to the damaged area. Once the pain has eased, gentle movement of the injured limb will keep the joint flexible and prevent muscle-wasting. For severe strains of the leg or arm muscles, it may be necessary to use a crutch or a sling for support. If the damage is severe, it may be necessary to consult a physiotherapist.

complementary treatments

Any of the following may help to speed up the healing process in a mild to moderate strain.

homeopathy

Bryonia This can be used after Arnica if a muscle strain is very much better for rest and considerably worse for even the slightest movement.

Ledum This can relieve muscle strains that feel cold internally but are soothed by bathing in cold water or a cool compress.

western herbalism

- Arnica cream can be immensely soothing when gently applied to a strain, especially it was the result of too much vigorous exercise after being unfit.

Warning Do not use Arnica on broken skin because it can trigger inflammation.

- Make a cool compress by freezing witch hazel in an ice-cube tray (taking care not to confuse these with regular ice cubes!). Wrap the cubes in a soft cloth and apply to the strained muscle.

sunburn/heatstroke

All of us run the risk of sunburn and/or heatstroke if we spend too much time in hot sunshine, especially if the humidity is high. However, the risk increases if we are very young or elderly because we become dehydrated more quickly. In their most severe form, both conditions are potentially very serious.

common symptoms

- **Rapid pulse**
- **Nausea**
- **Confusion**
- **Headache**

warning symptoms

Seek urgent medical attention if any of the following symptoms get worse or develop:

- **Rapid pulse**
- **Dizziness, disorientation and nausea**
- **High fever (40°C/102°F)**
- **Irritability and restlessness**
- **Drowsiness**
- **Dry, burning skin**
- **Changes in breathing patterns**
- **Headache**
- **Muscle cramps**
- **Collapse**

conventional treatments

Treatments focus on bringing down the temperature and rehydrating the body. For sunburn, creams will be necessary to soothe the skin. To avoid the problem recurring, extreme heat should be avoided in future.

complementary treatments

Very mild or minor episodes of sunburn or heatstroke should respond to the following measures. Should there be any sign of a more serious situation occurring, do not lose any time in getting emergency medical help.

aromatherapy

• For very mild sunburn, bathe in a coolish bath to which 10 drops of lavender oil have been added in order to help reduce inflammation and discomfort.

• Add 5 drops of lavender essential oil to 2 teaspoonsful of carrier oil and apply it gently to any hot, sore patches of skin.

homeopathy

Belladonna This is one of the first remedies to consider for mild classic sunburn with bright red patches of skin that radiate heat. Symptoms usually come on abruptly after over-exposure to sunlight and include a throbbing headache, with pains radiating from the top of the head.

Glonoin This remedy can help relieve symptoms of mild sunstroke with a severe headache where the pains are eased by bending the head backwards. As for Belladonna, symptoms usually come on strongly and quickly, and the skin feels generally hot and itchy.

Carbo vegetabilis (Carbo veg.) To relieve mild heatstroke and the exhaustion and fatigue that results from low-grade dehydration, try this remedy. Symptoms may include a craving for cool, fresh air, while being fanned and drinking plenty of fluids leads to a marked improvement.

Veratrum album Minor symptoms of heat exhaustion, with chills and feeling faint, are helped by this remedy. Although the skin feels hot, this is likely to alternate with shivering and a tendency to muscle cramps and there may be unquenchable thirst and a feeling of nausea.

naturopathy

Cooling down and rest is the first priority, as well as drinking to rehydrate the body. Loosen clothing and sponge the body with tepid water, or use a cool fan. Check the temperature regularly to make sure that it is within the normal range (36.5–37.5°C/97.7–99.5°F). If there is a low-grade headache, make the surroundings as open, cool and airy as possible. Rest is important to help the body get back on track, so peace and quiet are a priority.

• To soothe mild sunburn, apply cool natural yogurt to the affected skin. Use yogurt direct from the fridge for maximum calming effect.

western herbalism

• Dab on a solution of Urtica urens tincture (1 part tincture to 10 parts cooled, boiled water), followed by Urtica urens cream, to help calm down hot, stinging skin.

• Apply aloe vera juice or gel to soothe and take the heat out of localized areas of mildly sunburnt skin.

• Soothe minor sunburn by applying aloe vera gel or a diluted infusion of marigold (Calendula) flowerheads.

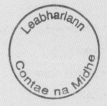

further reading

Blount, Trevor & **McKenzie**, Eleanor, *Pilates Basics*, Hamlyn, London, 2003

Curtis, Susan and **Fraser**, Romy, *Natural Healing for Women*, Thorsons, London, 2003

Lalvani, Vimla, *Complete Book of Yoga*, Hamlyn, London, 1999

MacEoin, Beth, *Natural Medicine*, Bloomsbury, London, 1999

Vyas, Bharti, *Beauty Wisdom*, Thorsons, London, 1997

Vyas, Bharti, *Fabulous Face*, Thorsons, London, 2002

Woodham, Anne and **Dr Peters**, David, *Encyclopedia of Complementary Medicine*, Dorling Kindersley, London, 1997

index

acknowledgements

Author acknowledgments:

During the course of writing this book, the following people have been immensely supportive, professional and kind, making the process of writing considerably more pleasurable. Jane McIntosh, Rachel Lawrance and Kate Tuckett at Hamlyn have been a delight to work with at every stage of the production of this book. Dr Paddy Gill must be singled out for special thanks and appreciation due her extremely prompt, constructive and impressive response when asked to comment on the conventional medical input in the text. Evelyn Miller provided very helpful conventional medical advice at very short notice, while my agent Teresa Chris must be sincerely thanked as always for all her excellent work in making all of this happen. And most of all, my love and thanks go as always, to my husband Denis. Without his inspiration, humour, and eagle-eyed proof reading skills I would feel quite lost.

Hamlyn acknowledgments:
Executive editor: Jane McIntosh
Senior editor: Rachel Lawrence
Executive art editor: Rozelle Bentheim
Designer: Geoff Borin
Illustrator: Nicola Gregory
Production controller: Manjit Sihra